THE MENOPAUSE
AND BEYOND

THE MENOPAUSE AND BEYOND

Sivalingam Nalliah

MBBS, MCGP, MRCOG, FRCOG, FAMM M Ed
Professor of Obstetrics and Gynecology
International Medical University Malaysia

To order additional copies of this book, contact:
Xlibris LLC
1-800-455-039
www.xlibris.com.au
Orders@xlibris.com.au
504213

CONTENTS

FOREWORD

'MENOPAUSE and BEYOND' is written for women who reach menopause. The author has been careful in having included several chapters dealing with various aspects of life after menopause. Emphasis is given to exercise, diet and relaxation apart from dealing in depth with effects of female hormones on the body.

The lay public has been exposed to the social media and to the medical fraternity to various views regarding the role of estrogen, progesterone and testosterone at menopause and beyond. There are differing levels of acceptance to advice and adherence to treatment in indicated cases.

Dr. Sivalingam has presented the facts surrounding the use of estrogen hormone therapy as he sees best without bias and discusses the overall impact in terms of benefits and risks.

Although this book is written for women in the menopausal years, it would also prove to be useful source of information for nurses and doctors who care for women as they grow older.

Tan Sri Dato (Dr) Abu Bakar Suleiman
Former Director General of Health
Ministry if Health
Malaysia.

ACKNOWLEGEMENT

I wish to express my gratitude to my wife Sivamani Rasiah and my two children Navin Anand and Vanitha Nandini who have supported and encouraged me to revise the original edition of this book which was written in 1996. An old teacher of mine, the late Professor N. Chandrasekaran needs mention as he volunteered to review the manuscript and gave me useful suggestions for improvement before his untimely demise.

I am indeed happy that there are excellent people at the International Medical University who have assisted me in getting some of the illustrations used in this book in time. To this end I must thank Aida Lina and Siti Aeysha. Apart from putting down in words my own experiences in managing women in the menopause for over 30 years, I went through several references for input and information. Many of the facts are drawn from the results of research done and published in medical journals and social media. I wish to thank all authors whose work I have quoted for sharing their research findings for the betterment of women's health and well being. There are too many for me to name them but I have indicated the sources I have used in both the Bibliography and in the text where relevant. Resources are often useful for readers to obtain up-to-date information regarding aging and management of menopause. I have included some of these where relevant.

I wish to thank open domains for the use of images of equipment and instruments that have been included in the text to make reading easier. I must particularly mention the following sources for some of the figures used in the book. They are of importance in attempting to explain difficult text based on human disease and I believe such data would be used for the betterment of women's health. The following sources are cited: Fig.6.4 (Snoots 3000), Fig.9.1 (Tufts' University), Table 10.3 (EEG, Lagopoulos), Fig. 20.1 (medical expo), Fig. 22.1 (smith-medical), Fig. 22.2 (Win-health), and Fig.22.3 (patient.uk.com).

Dr. Sivalingam Nalliah

PREFACE

'Menopause and Beyond' is a comprehensive account of aspects of life beginning from the transition phase a woman is in between 40-50 years and post-menopausal age. Increasing longevity of life to beyond seventy years of age means that women will spend a third of their life span after menopause. Planning for this stage of life is necessary so as to enjoy a good quality of life. Tremendous progress has been made in understanding the menopause and manifest bodily changes that follows after cessation of menstruation. Knowledge of the effects of oestrogen decline on the genital tract and various other parts of the body has enabled health caregivers to prescribe hormones, provide information on nutrition and other interventions for health and wellbeing. Currently most women know the beneficial effects of oestrogen on bone metabolism and atrophic vagina and also are aware of the correct indications for its use.

This book on menopause became a reality after seeing an increase in women seeking care as they grow older. Women are now forthcoming with complaints related to dry vagina, hot flashes, night sweats and urinary symptoms. Treating these ailments and disturbances improves quality of life. The chapters in the book attempts to answer as many questions as possible that may go through the mind of the menopausal woman.

The author has tried not to be biased in his views in use of oestrogen therapy and has drawn on current thoughts about benefits and controversies surrounding medical hormone therapy. Some of the comments are based on views expressed by professional bodies and consensus statements. Women should be well equipped with accurate information to make their own decisions and choices in selecting treatment options. Cultural and social influences also affect the attitudes and views of such decisions.

A variety of gynaecological and psychological disorders are seen in the older woman. Career change, retirement, relationship with family and bodily changes also impact on the woman's attitude to life after the menopause. Coping with internal conflicts and external stresses after the menopausal are not directly related to either aging or hormonal deprivation but that which comes with changed circumstances in family and society. Cognitive-behaviour therapy and counselling are used to tackle such problems in improving health and adapting to life during this stage.

As one grows older one would also succumb to age related diseases like hypertension, diabetes and obesity. Woman would be consulting a number of experts for each of the ailment. Taking control of her body and life hence involves deriving sufficient knowledge of both wellness and illness so that the woman stays in the driving seat in deciding best treatment options or combination of treatments with advice from health carers. Attention to good nutrition, regular exercise and management of stressors are equally important.

Sivalingam Nalliah

INTRODUCTION

In many ways the menopause appears to be the 'ragged' inverse image of menarche i.e the first menstrual cycle a women experiences in her life. The young adolescent starts menstruating around 10-12 years of age. She sprouts into womanhood through the influence of the hormones especially oestrogen. The vital female hormone begins to increase in its production as the ovaries come 'alive' from the time the girl is about 10 years old, influencing several target organs especially the female genital organs and the breasts. By the time she reaches 12 years of age, this powerful hormone exhibits it effect in an overt manner on the skin and breasts. As breasts develop, other visible changes occur in the young girl. Armpit hair and pubic hair development are easy to note. The gradual evolution of the uterus and vagina to prepare for the reproductive phase of life is eventually exhibited with the onset of regular menstruation.

Two hormones, oestrogen and progesterone, work in synchrony to carry through the reproductive capabilities for the next three or so decades in their own peculiar waxing and waning patterns. As the patient enters the mid-forties, a gradual decline in oestrogen levels become evident as the ovaries age and become atrophic. Bodily changes are gradual in onset with a transition phase beginning well before the recognition of menopause (the last menstrual cycle). The terms 'climacteric' or 'perimenopause' is use to describe this transition phase. Ovaries become functional in menarche but the opposite occurs in the perimenopausal period when the ovaries become senescent and exhaust themselves of 'eggs'. They 'shrivel' and stop producing adequate amounts of the female hormones, especially oestrogen.

Do we call the phase of life after menopause the end of the reproductive life or the beginning of a new phase of estrogen deficiency? Should we categorize the phase of life after the menopause a clinical entity that requires treatment as it is well recognised that physical and biochemical changes occur with ageing and there are observable manifestations related to the menopause? The genital organs 'flourished' under the influence of female hormones at puberty and thereafter but after the menopause the uterus shrinks and becomes smaller, menstruation halts and the bones become brittle. Oestrogen appeared to protect the woman during the reproductive age from heart disease but this no longer remains true after menopause. The prevalence of coronary heart disease catches up with that of men, age for age. However, a great number of women especially from Asia traditionally accept the changes that come with menopause as natural events and can't see what the fuss is about. Some find it disturbing in turning such a natural event into a disease that needs to be treated.

The phases of life in an adult woman

Final menstrual period (FMP)

Stages	−5	−4	−3	−2	−1	0	+1	+2
Terminology	Reproductive			Menopausal/Transition			Postmenopause	
	Early	Peak	Late	Early	Late*		Early*	Late
				Perimenopause				
Duration of stage	Variable			Variable		(a) 1 yr	(b) 4 yr	Until demise
Menstrual cycles	Variable to regular	Regular		Variable cycle length (>7 days different from normal)	>2 skipped cycles and an interval of amenorrhea (>60 days)	Amen −12 mo	None	
Endocrine	Normal FSH		↑ FSH	↑ FSH			↑ FSH	

Source: The Stages of Reproductive Aging Workshop (STRAW) staging system, Fertility and Sterility 76:874-878, 2001)

Advances in medicine led to a critical appraisal of hormones in the body and their relationship to functions. Endocrinologists and doctors interested in women's health now consider the oestrogen deficient state after the menopause as a treatable disease state. Hormone therapy appears to be appropriate to overcome the clinical manifestations due to oestrogen deficiency as oestrogen has been shown to be effective treating hot flashes and vaginal dryness. It appears to be a wonder drug in establishing a state of wellbeing, while protecting against bone loss and even coronary heart disease. This purported Robert A. Wilson to pen a book "Feminine Forever" in an effort to explain the possibility of women to lead an extended state of youthfulness for decades after the menopause.

Health managers are concerned about the immense cost involved in hospitalization, surgery and aftercare of bone fractures in older women as a result of osteoporosis, a treatable disease through use of oestrogen! From the economic point of view treatment of osteoporosis could reduce the prevalence of osteoporosis related fractures.

The miseries of menopause appear to rapidly disappear with restoration of oestrogen levels in the blood. Several claims that oestrogen replacement would also protect menopausal women against mental deterioration, mood swings and Alzheimer's disease was in vogue in the 1980s and 1990s but careful scientific evaluation suggests that this association is much more complicated to justify prescribing oestrogen. Positive effects on skin texture making it 'plump and moist' together with improvement of sexual function with application of oestrogen to the vagina have seen the increasing number of oestrogen preparations in the market.

Not all menopausal women elect to go on this hormone. In fact, when the use of oestrogen was at its height in the 1990's, less than 50% complied to long term therapy. The idea of being on a drug for several years does not appear acceptable to many. Attitudes to menopause vary between women and in different cultures. The spectre of cancer seems to halt prolonged oestrogen use. Are these risks real or imagined? Advocates of oestrogen therapy give conflicting views. 'Benefits outweigh risks' say many who are convinced that women will have a better quality of life with oestrogen.

The ultimate answer will lie on the wishes of the target population—menopausal women. Receptors on to which the oestrogen molecule docks in the body are found in over 300 different tissues. Current users of oestrogen and potential users should know about the wonders and risks of hormones prescribed in menopause. Where do the priorities lie? Is quality of life so badly affected that there is a need for oestrogen replacement? For instances, if hot flashes are incapacitating, there is a definite role for short term oestrogen therapy. In this context we are discussing a disease entity and not a phase of life. On the other hand, if the patient is a breast cancer survivor, alternatives to oestrogen may be preferred.

Counselling the menopausal woman on the various effects of menopause should be directed to bodily changes and the beneficial effects that oestrogen replacement has. Apart from focussing on oestrogen therapy directed counselling on avoiding obesity and attention to life style changes is essential. Smoking should cease and regular exercises are encouraged. Advice on nutrition, addressing stress factors and identifying depressive illness are Important for better health after the menopause.

Average Life Expectancy in Selected Countries

Country	Life Expectancy (years)
Hong Kong	82
Malaysia	74
USA	79
India	67.5
China	75
Japan	84
Sri Lanka	76
Thailand	74
Australia	82
Vietnam	73
Philippines	72

Source: The World: Life Expectancy (2013)

CHAPTER 1

HORMONES IN MENOPAUSE

In the 19th Century women rarely lived beyond the fifth decade of life. This scenario has changed rapidly. Current estimates indicate that women are living longer than men. In Malaysia the expected life span of women is 74.2 years. If the age of menopause is about 50 years of age, one can expect women to spend one third of their life span in the menopausal years.

The menopause is the eventual cessation of menstruation, an event that is clearly realized. The female child is born with about 400,000 follicles or potential eggs in the ovaries. However, not all will become functional. In fact only about 480 'eggs' are eventually released during the lifetime of the women after puberty. The follicular stimulating hormone (FSH) produced and stored in the brain (hypothalamus and pituitary) plays an active role in maturation of these 'eggs' each month. In human females, usually only one 'mature egg' is eventually released (ovulation) each month under the influence of another hormone called the luteinizing hormone (LH), also produced and released by the pituitary and hypothalamus. The remaining follicles that do not get recruited through the ensuing complex biochemical processes in the ovary become the 'corpus luteum' which produces progesterone. If the 'mature follicle' released by the ovary is fertilized by a sperm (in the fallopian tube), the lining of the uterus needs to be ready to receive the fertilized egg after a few days. The preparation of the uterine lining (endometrium) is completed by the progesterone that is released by the corpus luteum.

Hence two major hormones operate synchronously during the menstrual cycle to enable the uterus to eventually receive and grow the fertilized ovum. The dominant hormone during the first half of the menstrual cycle is oestrogen. After ovulation, progesterone becomes dominant as described above. The endometrium hence grows thicker under the influence of oestrogen and progesterone. Should pregnancy fail to occur, the corpus luteum shrivels, rarely lasting not more than 14 days? At the end of this period, if pregnancy fails to occur, menstruation will result from sloughing off the endometrial lining completing a 28 day menstrual cycle. The whole cycle is repeated the following month with follicular stimulating hormone recruiting a new cohort of 'follicles' for maturation and eventual release of one mature follicle at ovulation under the influence of luteinizing hormone. As one can see there is such fine synchrony between hormones FSH and LH produced by the pituitary glands acting on the ovaries and oestrogen and progesterone produced by the ovaries influencing the endometrium of the uterus to facilitate ovulation, fertilization and eventual implantation of the embryo in the uterus.

The menstrual cycle begins after menarche and continues till the end of reproductive life when menopause sets in at about 50 years of age. As the ovaries are endowed with a 'predetermined number of follicles 'at birth, follicles become depleted with each menstrual cycle. This explains the eventual loss of function of the ovaries at the end of the reproductive cycle leading life with an oestrogen depleted state after menopause.

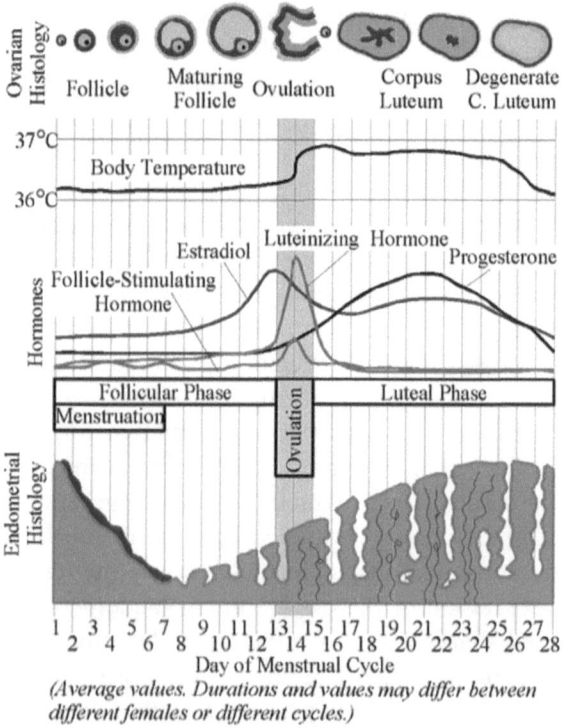

(Average values. Durations and values may differ between different females or different cycles.)

Fig. 1.1 Female hormones and the menstrual cycle

THE MENOPAUSE

The ovaries clearly are invested with a fixed number of potential follicles from birth and this declines in number as a woman ages after menarche. Each menstrual cycle depicts that pregnancy has not occurred with ultimate loss of a huge number of follicles. Hence with advancement of age approaching the menopause very few potential follicles remain. By the time a woman attains 50 years almost all the follicles are gone and the ovary becomes much smaller in size (ATROPHY OF THE OVARIES). Not much oestrogen is produced by the atrophic ovaries and hence has little or no effect on the lining of the uterus (endometrium). This culminates in cessation of menstruation and onset of menopause.

MENOPAUASE is derived from two words-MENO referring to month and PAUSE referring to cessation. Another term that often used synonymously is the CLIMATERIC. Menopause is a finite event, the age when menstruation stopped altogether referring to the last menstrual cycle. To achieve that event, several bodily changes and functionally changes occur. Other organs also show atrophic changes apart from the ovaries such as the vagina and urinary bladder. During the 'climacteric' which can cover a span of time ranging from 1-5 years around the menopause, the menstrual cycles become irregular and longer? Other functional disorders like excessive sweating and hot flashes may be evident. As these bodily changes are gradual in their onset many women tolerate symptoms related to the decline in oestrogen status and adapt well to the changing milieu.

Clearly, symptomatology varies from women to women and educational, cultural and socio-economic status impact on those who need specific treatment. The entire bodily changes and symptomatology realized by women prior to the onset of menopause is the 'climacteric'.

RECOGNIZING THE MENOPAUSE AND CLIMACTERIC

The 'climacteric' may not be easily recognized as functional and bodily changes are gradual. Many other life style changes occur during this time of a woman's life when children leave the home for education and career development. Relationship with her spouse may be affected by social circumstances and menopause itself. The 'empty nest syndrome' could invite depressive illness. Newly diagnosed medical illness like diabetes, hypertension, hypercholesterolemia and obesity can contribute to the need to alter lifestyle and depressive illness.

Functional changes that have been directed related to the climacteric and menopause need to exclude the effect of the factors mentioned so as to provide effective counselling and treatment.

The following have been clearly ascribed to menopause:

Early Menopausal Symptoms

    i.   VASOMOTOR INSTABILITY OR CLIMACTERIC SYMPTOMS

   ii.   PSYCHOSEXUAL DISTURBANCES

Late Menopausal Symptoms

   I.   OSTEOPOROSIS

  II.   CORONARY ARTERY DISEASE

Coronary heart disease cannot be said to be a consequence of menopause but women become susceptible to heart disease as much as men after the menopause. Late menopausal symptoms and psychosexual disturbances are discussed in other chapters.

VASOMOTOR INSTABILITY is a high sounding word. It is said to be a consequence of depletion of oestrogen in the body during the climacteric. Of great prominence in this condition is the embarrassing spells of HOT FLASHES (FLUSHES) and NIGHT SWEATS. These are often associated with irritability and sleep disturbances.

With declining oestrogen levels in the climacteric many women experience hot flashes. It is estimated that 75% of women in the West experience this symptom. In about 80 % hot flashes prevail for about a year and may remain for up to 5 years in about 25 % of these women if untreated. It is not uncommon to experience hot flashes prior to the cessation of menstruation.

The first indication of a hot flash is a sensation of pressure headache. Palpitations, which are the awareness of one's heart beating, may also be noticed. The flash itself is described as a wave of hot sensation beginning in the head and extending to the upper chest and arm. Some women feel it in the entire body. Associated with this feeling of 'heat' comes sweating. In most instances hot flashes come in episodes and may last from one to several minutes. It is surmised that certain chemicals in the brain (central transmitters) influence both temperature control and release of gonadotropic releasing hormones in the brain. These biochemical changes appear to be a result of sudden decline in oestrogen production in the ovaries.

Hot flashes at night with sweating are associated with SLEEP DISTURBANCE. Night sweat can be extremely disturbing. The quality of sleep one gets influences how we perform the next day. Irritability and fatigue are common if we do not get a reasonable amount of sound sleep.

Several central nervous system symptoms related to oestrogen deficiency have been reported in the menopause. These include nervousness, anxiety, and depression, alteration of sensory perception and loss of balance.

Since the events leading to the menopause are gradual in onset, it may be difficult to make a clear diagnosis and ascribe it to oestrogen deficiency. Talking to the patient to elicit an accurate history and examining her so as to exclude other disease states is essential. Hot flashes and night sweats are classical manifestations of oestrogen deficiency. Changes in menstrual cycle which often leads to infrequent cycles with less flow amount and vaginal dryness are often due to the menopause.

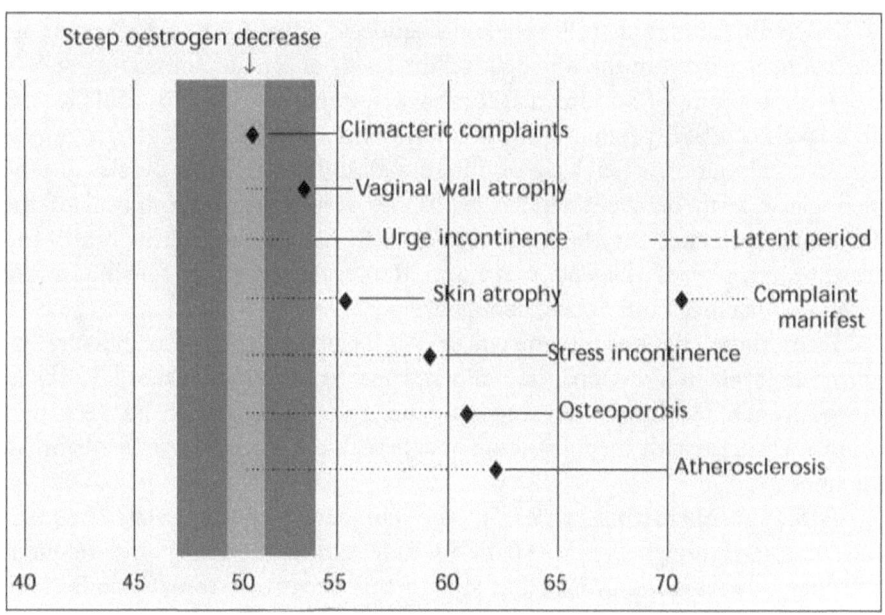

Figure 1.2 Age of onset of bodily changes following menopause

MENSTRUAL BLEEDING

Menstrual bleeding occurs because of interplay of hormones produced in the brain and ovaries in a well synchronised way. FSH, LH, oestrogen and progesterone have specific role in the process. When menstruation occurs in humans it indicates that pregnancy did not occur if the patient has had coitus. FSH facilitates the recruitment of a number of follicles in the ovary to begin maturing but ultimately only one follicle eventually reaches a state of maturation reaching the surface of the ovary. A surge of LH from the brain is required for the mature follicle to escape out of the ovary so as to be picked up by the finger like 'fimbriae' of the fallopian tube. The mature follicle then travels down the fallopian tube to be fertilized by a sperm (if coitus had taken place). During the recruitment and maturation process a complex series of hormones are produced in the cells of the ovaries which include oestrogen and progesterone.

Active changes in the endometrium of the uterus occur under the dominant influence of oestrogen in the first half of the menstrual cycle and in the second half of the menstrual cycle, under progesterone effect. Menstruation occurs at the end of a 28 day (normal) cycle should a pregnancy not occur.

Increasing levels of oestrogen turn off further release of FSH and LH by the brain through a well-executed 'feedback system'. Should there be no ovulation, as is seen in the menopause; the levels of female hormones are very low with a failure of an effective feedback system. This would result is very high levels of FSH (produced in the brain) with levels of 35-40 IU/L.

A combination of a lack of functional follicles in the ovaries in the menopause with deficient female hormones results in a withdrawal of the hormonal influence on the endometrium (lining of the uterine wall) and eventual atrophy of the endometrium. Menstruation is not possible under such circumstances and hence menopause occurs.

From these changed circumstances it is clear that if one was measure the hormone levels in a menopausal women, the FSH level will exceed 35 IU/L, the oestrogen levels will be very low and endometrium will be very thin when measured with an ultrasound machine measuring less than 4 mm in thickness.

Although menstrual cycles in the climacteric become less frequent and flow is diminished, some patients may experience heavy and frequent bleeding. This is not common but should this occur the woman should seek medical consultation for evaluation and treatment. Some pathology in the uterus may be present masquerading as abnormal bleeding in the menopausal years. It is mandatory for the uterine cavity to be evaluated by looking within the cavity using a hysteroscopy and /or taking a scraping (biopsy) of the uterine lining with a suitable device. Tumours of the uterine lining include endometrial hyperplasia, endometrial polyps and even endometrial cancer.

Postmenopausal Bleeding

Women should not bleed from the genital tract after attaining menopause. Any form of bleeding, no matter how trivial requires a medical consultation. As some women close to the menopause have irregular and prolonged menstrual cycles, they may be confused as to when POSTMENOPAUSAL BLEEDING is present. To avoid this confusion, conventionally a doctor's opinion is not required till six months has passed since the last menstrual bleeding in women in the climacteric. Once we clearly comprehend the functions of the ovaries and their hormonal control together with how the latter exert their effect on the endometrium of the uterus one could conclude that any bleeding after six months of the last menstrual period in women between 45-55 is abnormal. A general rule of thumb is to seek medical consultation if 'menstrual bleeding 'is abnormal after the age of 40 years.

Causes of Postmenopausal Bleeding

There may be several reasons for abnormal bleeding after the menopause. Some may be due to disease while others may be induced by medication. The following are the common conditions:

  i.   Atrophic vaginitis
 ii.   Hormone Therapy (Oestrogen)
iii.   Benign tumours of the endometrium and cervix
 iv.   Malignant tumours of the genital tract
  v.   Local injury to the genital tract like vaginal trauma

After the menopause oestrogen deprivation results in thinning and shrivelling of the tissues of the genital tract and urinary bladder. Apart from thinning and atrophy, vaginal lubrication is minimal and it becomes narrowed causing pain during sexual intercourse. Minor trauma as a result of cleaning the vaginal with tissue paper can cause slight bleeding. This is due to ATROPHIC VAGINITIS which is best treated with application of oestrogen creams for about two weeks.

Women who have been prescribed hormone therapy with oestrogen and progestogen on a cyclic basis will bleed from the uterine cavity after the hormones are stopped at the end 3 weeks in a four week cycle (WITHDRAWAL BLEEDING). Counselling is essential before initiating hormone therapy about withdrawal bleeding and side-effects.

In the absence of atrophic vaginitis and withdrawal bleeding following hormone therapy, one needs to evaluate the women by performing a gynaecological examination to ensure she does not suffer from the other conditions listed above. Non-malignant conditions like cervical and endometrial polyps need to be surgically removed. More sinister conditions like endometrial and cervical cancer may present as irregular 'menstrual 'bleeding. A definite diagnosis needs to be clinched before the woman is dismissed as normal variant of bleeding in the climacteric.

Conclusion

Pituitary hormones, oestrogen and progesterone play vital roles in the regulation of the reproductive system in women. The female genital tract is designed to enable the uterus to carry a pregnancy to term. When pregnancy does not occur menstruation will follow. Cycle menstruation is affected with declining oestrogen and atrophy of the ovaries. A sound knowledge of the complex relationship between female hormones and the genital tract would empower woman to know her bodily functions and better prepare her for the effects of menopause. Bleeding from the genital tract after six months of the menopause is abnormal and would require a medical consultation. As both benign and malignant tumours of the genital tract occur in the climacteric investigations are indicated.

CHAPTER 2

MENOPAUSE THE WORLD OVER

Aristotle, the Greek philosopher, mentions that the menopause occurs at 50 years of age in 322 BC. In 1729, John Friend reduced this number to 49 years and recent studies have not differed much from these historical figures. Ever since menopause has been recorded as an important biological event in a woman's life, there have been records of associated disturbances in other functions of the body. In most countries the menopause occurs between 48-52 years with an average age of 50. Uncommonly, the menopause has been seen in younger women. When it occurs below 40 years of age the term PREMATURE MENOPAUSE is used. On the other hand most women should have attained menopause by the age of 55 years. Robert Wilson wrote in 1966 about hormonal changes that takes place around the menopause 'that kindled worldwide interest' in various treatment strategies. The cultural context within which a woman lives has a significant impact on her perspectives of climacteric symptoms and life after the menopause.

From the medical aspect, one can recognise various disturbances in the functions of the human body even before the onset of menopause. Some of these have been mentioned in the previous chapter. Most of these symptoms are amenable to treatment with estrogen hormone. However, from cultural aspects, different views are expressed. Cross-cultural analysis of the menopause and its related disorders indicate different attitudinal approaches. Asians appear to be different from Europeans in accepting the symptoms of the menopause. The level of literacy varies in different populations and impacts on the frequency of medical consultations.

Before some of the differences and similarities are discussed, it would be prudent to recapitulate some of the common symptoms associated with the menopause.

Symptoms of Menopause

Without getting into specific details, some symptoms come early in life before the cessation of menstruation (menopause), whilst others are much more delayed in their onset. We will try to look at the variance in symptomatology in different parts of the world.

1. Vasomotor symptoms

Up to 80% of Dutch women suffer from hot flashes while the Mayan women of Mexico do not report such symptoms. This may be due the acceptance of hot flashes as a normal phase of ageing. There is also a possibility that women may not volunteer this information a disabling phenomenon. Access to healthcare may be a factor to consider too. The Rajput women if North India, apparently receive hot flashes positively as being rewarding enabling them to participate in the daily activities with the menfolk!. Japanese women, on the other hand, do not place great significance on the menopause. Hot flashes were not a prominent disorder Malaysia, Indonesia and the Philippines. In many countries the quality of life is not severely affected when the menopause is well accepted culturally as a new phase of life beyond the reproductive years. Cultural acceptance of the menopause may suppress symptoms like hot flashes, night's sweats and mood swings, passing them off as normal variants of life. A study on 400 Chinese workers in Hong Kong by G. Tang revealed few complained of hot flashes and psychological symptoms.

Literacy impacts on symptomatology as is seen in Asian women. Higher literacy is associated with access to healthcare. Hence, the more educated a woman is, the greater the chance of medical consultations for menopausal symptoms. This has been reported in Malaysia and other Asian women.

2. Sexual Practices

In many Asian countries including India, Thailand, Pakistan, Malaysia and Indonesia, sexual desires and sexual activity waned with the onset of menopause. Moderate to severe atrophy and shrivelling of the vagina and urinary bladder were common in over 50% of women in the menopause. With inherent changed attitude towards sex at the menopause together with genital tract atrophy, the desire for sexual activity would invariably be less frequent. With due modesty given to matters related to sexual activity and the reluctance to vaginal examination, the Malaysian woman adopts a more conservative attitude. This is especially so in among rural women who take on the role of child minding in extended families. Information related to sexual activity often is not volunteered in medical consultations. More research is wanton in this area and population based studies should incorporate socio-economic and cultural practices in elucidating attitudes to sexual practices in both urban and rural areas.

Heath care providers need communication skills to elicit such history from clients with an intention to both gather more data and also empower women to take make informed choices so as improve quality of life. Age, educational level and attitudes to treatment of symptoms related to menopause need to be factored into data analysis. A global study in 2005 involving 26,000 adults aged 40-80 in 29 countries was revealing. Sexual difficulties are evident in the older adults worldwide. In terms of a lack of sexual interest women in the US had higher rates than European women (33% vs., 27%). The rates were lower in women of East Asia (35%), Southeast Asia (43%) and Middle East (43%). Attitudes to sexuality, discomfort during sex, body image and lack of interest appear to be seen in women worldwide.

3. Smoking

Smoking has many bad effects on the body including an increased incidence of lung ailments and coronary heart disease. Women who smoke tend to reach menopause 1.5 years earlier than non-smokers. Smoking is prevalent in the West and is increasing rapidly in Asia. Great harm is seen when more than 10 sticks are smoked regularly each day. It has been reported that women who smoke will experience hot flashes to a greater degree together with sleep disturbances compared to non-smokers.

Osteoporosis is also more pronounced in smokers. Hip fractures after a fall is higher in postmenopausal women. It appears that for every 5 years a woman smokes the risk of a hip fracture increase 6%. This figures drops three fold if a woman has stopped smoking for about 15 years prior to menopause.

4. Urinary and Bowel Problems in Menopause

Leakage of urine while coughing and inability to control the urinary bladder while attempting to reach the toilet are not uncommon urinary problems in older women. These are called urinary stress incontinence and overactive bladder respectively. Details appear in Chapter 20. Urinary tract infection requiring menopausal woman to go to the toilet more frequently are also common in the menopause. Many of the urinary symptoms are related to estrogen deficiency and its effect on the collagen supporting the neck and walls of the urinary bladder and its outlet. Inability to control 'wind' and constipation may also occur in this period of transition.

Weaknesses in the support of the female genital organs result in various degrees of relaxation of the organs. The atrophic uterus could prolapse and so could the vagina and rectum. The patient initially may feel a sense of 'something' coming down and later realize the prolapse of the genital organs. Weight gain and obesity are also common in the older woman and contributes to genital organ prolapse.

Both urinary problems and genital prolapse are common worldwide and frequently require specific treatment.

5. Acceptance of Specific Treatment

Cultural practices and personal attitudes to menopause influence, to a large extent, treatment with hormones, surgery for genital organ prolapse and urinary stress incontinence and obesity. Strengthening the vagina with Kegel's exercise requires adherence to treatment and patience. Hormone therapy has become controversial over the last decade since concerns of breast cancer has been reported with long term use of specific types of estrogen and progestogen in the Women's Health Initiative data analysis in 2002 in the US. The current opinion that hormone therapy has benefits in relieving menopausal symptoms and also bladder problems when used appropriately under the supervision of a doctor needs sufficient counselling.

The introduction of bio-identical medication and alternative medicine for improving symptoms of menopause now increases treatment options. The provision of accurate information of the value of hormone treatment, use of alternatives and benefits of non-pharmacologic strategies varies from country to country and can be confusing to the lay public. Health care givers need to play an integral role in identifying the symptoms clients have so that specific and safe treatment may be provided bearing in mind cost of such treatment and side effects.

Withdrawal bleeding while being prescribed cyclical hormones in the menopause may be startling to women who had not been forewarned of the return of 'menstruation' leading to non-adherence to treatment. Alternative treatment like the 'no-bleed' regime should be better in such patients where there is a benefit of use. Many Muslim and Hindu women in Malaysia prefer the non-bleed regime as it would not interfere with their religious routines and visit to places of worship. On the other hand women who prefer the cyclical regime where they get their monthly bleeds prefer the 'drug free' week and may accept the 'nuisance of the menstrual bleeding'.

6. Information on Menopause

Women in this transition phase of life should be given sufficient information on both the natural processes involved in the climacteric and treatment options for better decision making. This should be the responsibility of health providers as information from friends; internet and the media may not be sufficiently clear or accurate. General practitioners, gynaecologist and 'well woman' clinic care providers can assess the patient's symptoms and suggest appropriate treatment. As a host of complaints are seen as one ages, it would require an expert to make an accurate diagnosis.

Opportunistic screening is now commonplace as part of 'well women' clinics worldwide especially among the affluent. Screening for breast disease and genital tract cancers would involve intimate examination of the breast for lumps and pap smears following vaginal examination. Such examination requires explanation and the value of such assessments so as not to alarm women. Breast examination for lumps is not sensitive and small tumours cannot be picked up. This must be made known to the woman. Routine blood tests for cancer screening are usually not encouraged though mammograms may be done after the age of 50 years. Cost of investigations needs to be borne in mind and be kept to the minimum.

Counsellors who may be nurses and medical personnel require sufficient skills and keep abreast of current medical literature on controversies surrounding hormone treatment of menopausal symptoms and the effectiveness of alternative medicine including medication and acupuncture. Engagement in good dialogue with clients could promote positive approaches to life style changes and personal health after the menopause with less reliance on hormone therapy as the sole treatment strategy. Where treatment with specific therapy is indicated health care givers should develop individualised programs for women taking into consideration the woman's educational, cultural and religious background. Where a hormone of other medication is essential for symptom control, the most cost-effective medication is selected.

It is generally agreed that where menopausal symptoms like hot flashes and nights sweats are extremely disabling estrogen therapy for short duration of 1-2 years is excellent for relieve of symptoms provided there are no contraindications for the use of estrogen.

Busy doctors and health care givers may not spend enough time exploring the health and psychological problems of menopausal women. Adequate counselling requires sufficient time and sympathetic listening ears. If the information given on the first consult is inadequate repeat consultations are in order so as to be sufficiently furnished with all essential information before beginning specific medical treatment.

Conclusion

The age of attaining menopause has been constant over hundreds of years. It appears to be similar the world over. Cigarette smokers appear to reach menopause earlier than non-smokers and are also at a higher risk of osteoporotic hip fractures.

Although 25 % of women do not suffer from menopausal symptoms a good proportion of women with severe symptoms benefit from hormone treatment. Asian women appear to be less disturbed by disabling menopausal symptoms like psychosexual problems and hot flashes. Socio-cultural practices may be influencing factors.

With increasing life span of women, long term complications following menopause like osteoporosis and coronary heart disease will be more prevalent in most countries throughout the world. There is a need for individualization of treatment which would include both medication and life style changes.

CHAPTER 3

THE MENOPAUSE AND CLIMACTERIC
-Coping with a new phase of life

The menopause is an important event in a woman's life. The PERIMENOPAUSAL PERIOD is a phase of life that surrounds the menopause when both functional and bodily changes are experienced for a few years before the menopause and immediately after, the CLIMACTERIC. Dr, John Stud, a prominent gynaecologist from the UK stated that the menopause should be considered 'BIOLOGICAL SABOTAGE' because of the multi-system disorders it causes. Robert Wilson, an American gynaecologist was 'vilified' by both the press and the medical profession in the 1960s for suggesting women be maintained on hormones in his book, 'Feminine Forever'.

While the medical profession looks at symptoms and effects of the menopause as an endocrine disorder which can be salvaged with hormone therapy, the general population often has differing views. Cross-cultural differences, religious views and adequate knowledge of the transition from late reproductive stage in the 40s to menopause and beyond influences treatment strategies of symptoms.

Why is discussion on the menopause and post menopause so prominent now?

Menopause and medical hormone treatment have become prominent since the 70s though the menopause has been known as a distinct state

---

from the times of the Greeks. Why has this phenomenon captured the eyes of women today? Medical advances have made it possible to understand the role of hormones in general and female hormones, in particular much better. It is possible to measure the hormones of the body from blood tests. We can now relate the functions of hormones to bodily changes. We can clearly state that many symptoms that women suffer around the time of menopause is related to decline in estrogen. With advanced technology available today it is possible to precisely determine the role played by the hypothalamus and pituitary in the brain. We have detailed knowledge of the functioning of the ovaries and the specific roles played by estrogen, progesterone, androgen and variety of other hormones influencing the reproductive system. Molecular biology has advanced so much that it is possible to use various types of 'probes' to outline molecular pathways and the way receptors work. The hormone status of the women through her menstrual cycle has been worked out with a clear knowledge of fluctuations of the female hormones during the cycle. Some psychological and physical experiences women have during the menstrual cycle are related to these fluctuations. The ability to establish hormone profiles in women not only has been useful in understanding and treating menopausal symptoms but has also been valuable in treating menstrual disorders and infertility.

The improvement in living conditions worldwide has enabled humans to survive longer with life expectancy of women in developing countries going beyond 70 years. Although the age of menopause has not changed (48-52 years) women are living for about 20-30 years beyond menopause. That means women now live a third of their life span after menopause. The medical fraternity has been studying the implications of living beyond menopause in a state of estrogen deprivation and attempting to develop ways and means in maintaining a good quality of life based on prevention and treatment of specific disorders and disturbances experienced by post-menopausal women. Osteoporosis, hot flashes, dry vagina, urinary symptoms are some of such conditions that are amenable to treatment. Most menopausal symptoms are due to ovaries ceasing to function after an average age of 50 years. The decline in ovarian function is a slow one running over 4-5 years. The physical and functional changes women experience is subtle and silent. Clinical manifestations like hot flashes and night sweats are not experienced by all women. It appears to be more apparent in educated women rather than those in lower socio-economic groups. Bone loss is silent event that may not be recognised unless the woman has a fracture of the bone after a fall or becomes 'bent double' over the spine. Changes in breast tissue, dry skin and vagina take time to develop. Atrophic vagina is experienced after some months to years of menopause. Medical disorders like coronary heart disease and strokes are more evident in the older woman. The protective role of estrogen on the heart and blood vessels is now realised as the incidence of myocardial infarction parallels that of men after menopause.

How do women respond to the menopause?

Since specific symptoms related to menopause are recognised several months and years prior to the event, women vary in their complaints. Bone loss declines after 35 years of age but becomes more evident closer to menopause. Yet it may not produce any symptoms. Vasomotor symptoms like hot flashes can be short lived in some lasting for about 6 months but can be felt by others for as long as two years. Table 3.1 shows the common health problems of women after menopause.

Table 3.1 Health Problems of Post-Menopause

Early Onset	
Central Nervous System	Hot flashes Night Sweats Headaches Palpitations
Skin	Dryness Thinning Dry hair Brittle nails
Uro-genital	Dry vagina Painful Intercourse Urinary disturbances
Psychological	Irritability Mood swings Inability to concentrate Decreased libido
Late Onset	
Coronary heart disease	Ischemic heart disease, Myocardial infarction, death
Osteoporosis	Low backache, bone fractures, loss of height

Changes in the woman's body and symptomatology depend on the rate at which the ovaries 'age' over the perimenopausal years and consequent decline in estrogen. Symptoms like hot flashes and night sweats are immediate in susceptible women after surgical removal of the both ovaries.

Women's response to estrogen deprivation is also related to her ability to adjust to this 'major change in life'. Cultural factors and acceptance of menopause as normal phase of life makes it easier for many woman to live with little disturbance in quality of their lives. Psychological symptoms and attitudes to sexual activity are at great variance in women from different ethnic groups and geographical regions. Many women accept menopause as a passing phase and get on with life as best suits them. Muscle aches and back pain may be ascribed and accepted as part of aging. Decrease in frequency of sexual intercourse can be due to decreased sexual desire, again accepted as part of growing old. Disability in the spouse and painful intercourse because of atrophic vaginitis are reasons that coitus no longer becomes a 'need'.

Long terms effects of estrogen depletion such as bone loss and the cardiovascular disease may be not be realized due to the silent nature of its onset especially osteoporosis and coronary heart disease which are accepted as events of old age.

Coping with menopause

The menopause is a finite event i.e cessation of menstruation; it will occur in all menstruating women at about 50 years of age. The onset is earlier if surgery is done with removal of the uterus and /or ovaries. While estrogen decline is rapid after surgical removal of both ovaries, women who have ovaries preserved at hysterectomy before the natural onset of menopause tend to develop menopausal symptoms about two years prior to natural menopause. In some women the ovaries fail to function and menstruation cease before the age of 40 years (PREMATURE MENOPAUSE) and will benefit from medical hormone therapy.

Estrogen therapy has a value in many instances as quality of life and wellbeing improves. However, many other events in life affect our behaviour as we grow older. Loss of a loved one, children growing up and leaving home, change of career and early retirement are all factors that will affect both psychological health and adaptation to changing environment. Hormone therapy would not be able to address all aspects and disorders seen in post menopause. Adaptation to changes in life should be aligned to cultural and religious views and personal perspectives. Four strategies worthy of mention apart from what has been mentioned are:

1. Good nutrition

2. Rest and relaxation
3. Exercise
4. (Medical Hormone Therapy)

Each of these is discussed in subsequent chapters.

How does one predict menopause?

Although most women attain menopause around 50 years of age, some experience it earlier while other reach it later. Cessation of menstruation for a year is a definable sign. As the females hormones decline the duration of menstrual flow become less, menstrual cycles decrease in frequency and eventually cease.

Three predictors are:

- Menstrual cycles become less in number and irregular
- Duration of menstrual flow decreases in amount per cycle (less and lighter)
- Hot flashes and night sweats

Mood swings, ease of irritability and depressive feelings cannot be directly attributed to estrogen decline as many social and environmental factors need to be explored for such feelings. Dry vagina and atrophic vaginitis are not predictive as they are experienced some months to years after onset of menopause. Brittle bone and coronary heart disease are both late onset events.

Do all postmenopausal women require estrogen?

Scientific knowledge has linked estrogen deprivation to a number of correctable bodily changes like osteoporosis and atrophic vaginitis. It would be wrong to deny the beneficial effects of hormone therapy if there is an indication.

Beneficial effects of estrogen therapy

Short term

- Relieves hot flashes and night sweats
- Decreases vaginal dryness and irritation
- Permits comfortable sexual intercourse

Long Term

- Prevents bone loss
- Reduces risk of heart disease if given within 10 years of menopause (50-59 years)

Estrogen (with/without progestogen) was very popular as it had immense beneficial effects on many of the complaints related to the menopause till the results of scientific studies (WHI 2002 & 2004) cautioned its use linking to slight increase in breast cancer, stroke and cardiovascular disease though there were clear evidence of the benefit on prevention of bone loss and reduction in colon cancer. The sudden decline in use of estrogen (with/ without progestogen) also saw a decline in the incidence of invasive breast cancer in the UK.

As more information is available over the years physicians are clearer about when and how to prescribe estrogen (with/without progestogen). Many of these findings are discussed later in the book. For a full description on current indications and guidelines on use of medical hormone therapy, the reader should refer to Royal College of Obstetricians and Gynaecologists (UK) Greentop Guidelines on Hormone Therapy and North American Menopause Society Guidelines.

Taking estrogen and progestogen on a long term basis would require close monitoring for good and non-beneficial effects. Women desirous of taking medical hormone therapy should have sufficient information and weigh the benefits and risks when making decisions. Hot flashes and night sweats respond very well with estrogen therapy and so do vaginal atrophy. As these conditions do not need very long term use of hormones adherence to prescription is high. However, some reports state that when estrogen therapy is prescribed only 40 % comply with the duration advised. On the other hand, there are contraindications to taking hormones. Some of them are real because the risks are too high such as those who have been diagnosed with breast cancer. In others the contraindications are not 'absolute' such as high blood pressure, diabetes mellitus and liver disease. Your doctor would explain if the hormone can be taken or if some alternative formulations are preferred like application to the skin rather than taking the hormone orally.

Breast cancer in women is by the most worrisome in any discussion on the association with estrogen with/without progestogen therapy. The breast tissue is sensitive to estrogen and progestogen and new knowledge explains the processes involved as to how specific tissues in the breast behave in the presence of naturally produced female hormones and also with use of specific formulations used in medical hormone therapy. Current guidelines in use of estrogen hormones and alternatives like bio identical hormones address these issues so as to keep women informed on safe use of medical hormone therapy.

The effect estrogen have on the lining of the uterus (endometrium) has been well addressed in scientific studies. Unopposed (i.e sole use) estrogen without adding progestogen for about 12-14 days in a cycle will eventually lead to new growths in the uterus which ranges from polyps in the endometrium to excessive proliferation and endometrial cancer. The guidelines in hormone therapy are now clear that addition of progestogen protects the endometrium when estrogen is taken.

Women who attain menopause early (premature menopause i.e. before 40 years) benefit from a combination of estrogen and progestogen therapy. They would have 'menstrual bleeding' monthly in a 21 day regime and the treatment improves quality of life and prevents the early onset of osteoporosis. There is a protective effect on heart and blood vessels. A similar approach may be taken if a woman has had surgical removal of both ovaries at an early age because of benign gynaecological disease. The duration of treatment and when hormones should be stopped should be discussed with the attending physician.

How long should women taken estrogen therapy

Estrogen is prescribed for specific purposes in women who fulfil the criteria for medical hormone therapy. Many factors will help decide as to how long women should take medical hormone therapy. As discussed above, if premature menopause is present she could be on the medication till the age of natural menopause. On the other hand a 70 year old woman would have more risks than benefits in taking estrogen for a long period and this is shown in the WHI study where there is an increased risk, albeit small, of breast cancer, coronary heart disease, stroke and deep vein thrombosis with a combination of estrogen and progestogen (the study uses a particular formulation of estrogen and progestogen). However, if the main problem is atrophic vaginitis the use of local application of estrogen is acceptable.

A practical approach would be to screen women for risks of common diseases like invasive breast cancer, osteoporosis, heart disease, stroke and deep vein thrombosis. The age of the woman, her weight and reasons for hormone therapy are then factored in. When all these variables are considered then a plan can be drawn as to what preparation of hormone is best for the woman, what regime suits her and how long she should be on the hormones. Younger women who have attained menopause well before 50 years would certainly benefit from hormone treatment and derive the benefits mentioned including prevention of bone loss.

Loss of bone is maximal during the first 10 years of menopause. After that there is slowing because of aging. Current views are that estrogen should not be prescribed for osteoporosis but only for prevention of the condition. There is several specific 'bone enhancing' medication like alendronate that have no adverse effects of estrogen and is best used for osteoporosis (see chapter 6). Few women beyond 60 are candidates for long term estrogen therapy. The aim is to treat specific complaints like dry vagina and urinary, if present.

Conclusion

The menopause and the period around it (perimenopausal) are associated directly and indirectly with many body functions. The brain, heart, bones, genital organs, skin and urinary bladder are affected at some stage. These changes clearly are related to estrogen deprivation with atrophy of the ovaries. A simple solution would be to supplement estrogen. This was the practice in 1980s and 90s till scientific studies cautioned the widespread use of medical hormone therapy. The benefits of estrogen on the genital tract and bone are well understood. Concerns on effect of estrogen and progestogen on the breast have assisted medical practitioners to draw clear guideline on their use so as to make it safe for women. The public need to be kept informed on new developments with more research findings from on-going clinical and experimental studies.

Patient's views on how she is coping with symptoms of menopause and what her views are about medical hormone therapy is paramount in decision making. Cultural and religious views need to be factored in when making choices in medial hormone therapy. Hormone therapy is but one aspect of caring for women past the menopause. Life style changes, exercise, nutrition are equally important in improving quality of life.

CHAPTER 4

PSYCHOLOGICAL ASPECTS OF MENOPAUSE

Edward John Tilt, a physician in Brighton, England was the first person to write in the English Language on the psychological problems associated with menopause in his book, 'The Change of Life in Health and Disease' published in 1857. Although much research has been done on the psychological aspects of menopause, it has become difficult to summarily state that particular psychological symptoms are directly related to the menopause because of the difficulties encountered in defining certain symptoms specific to this period in life.

Psychological symptoms expressed by women in the West are different from that in the East with culture and beliefs impacting on clinical manifestations. Literacy, education and social strata and awareness of menopausal symptoms impacts on women seeking treatment.

Psychological and emotional symptoms are common around the menopause, but the causes are complex. Anxiety, depression, sadness, difficulty concentrating, overreacting to minor upsets, anger and irritability, forgetfulness and mood swings are all typical psychological problems. Hormonal changes are thought to be responsible for a proportion of these symptoms, but it is hard to be certain which symptoms are hormonal in origin, and which are due to other changes in a woman's life around that time. Studies indicate that many cases of depression, for example, relate more to personal circumstances than to the menopause itself. Studies have also indicated that women who are generally happy with their lives experience fewer problems during menopause.

Many situations and personal events affect the lives of women past 40-50 years. Children begin leaving home for education and starting their own families, retirement with consequent changed lifestyle, personal ailment and that of surviving parents will take a toll on personal freedom with possible financial implications. Changes in personal habits and occupation of spouse could affect the woman. Widowhood is a yet another possibility that affects psychological state.

Obesity and chronic illness like hypertension, diabetes mellitus and even stroke can have severe effects. Physical ageing with need for assisted living are situations that can result in loss of self-image and low self-esteem.

Hot flashes and night sweats disturb sleep pattern and causes embarrassment and irritability. Other menopausal symptoms like dry vagina could be reasons for not having coitus which in turn can affect intimacy and self-worth.

How are concepts of life viewed during this period of life? Is it acceptable to have sexual intercourse past the age of menopause? Is it taboo to discuss intimate sexual health in this phase of life? Many of such questions are not discussed openly as women have their own views as to how socially acceptable it is to discuss matters related to feelings and mental health. The spouse plays a role in the equation. He would also have views and will have to contend with his own views of life in old age, his needs and likes about sexual health and personal needs. Is depression an issue in him, is he actively in employ, does he suffer any age related ailments that impacts on personal relationship with his wife? How is the relationship working when both parties are at home? What are their engagements and how do both relate to family and friends? What new hobbies have been adopted and how is time spent in retirement? As one can see, immense psychological and social adaptation is prevalent and need to be tackled effectively to lead a stress free life.

Sickness and ailments negatively impact on mental health. As one grows older, diabetes, hypertension, stroke and obesity are seen in increasing rates. Arthritis can be disabling and painful knees due to osteoarthritis would require special care and perhaps surgery with knee replacement. Falls in the menopause women can result in fractures especially when osteoporosis has set in. This can result in prolonged hospitalization and disability contributing to depression and loss of mobility.

When depression in the menopause is discussed, one needs to distinguish the physical disablement and disease from psychological problems attributed to menopause per se. Cancer in old age has severe psychological effect arising from discovery of the disease and feeling of helplessness arising from the treatment given by way of radical surgery, chemotherapy and radiation therapy. The combined effect can be devastating.

As one can surmise it becomes difficult to ascribe changes in mood and behaviour in the post-menopausal years to estrogen deficiency alone! Life style changes and adjustment to changing circumstances are important. The appropriate adaptation to changed family situation helps immensely in overcoming stress and improves psychological wellbeing.

It is said that 'total life stress' peaks in early menopause and that is also the time when psychological symptoms are reported in many women. It has been conclusively shown that 'exit stress' are of particular importance. Exit stresses included loss of a partner and loss of role as a leader in the family.

Sleep deprivation due to night sweats and getting up frequently at night will have its effect the following morning. Quality sleep and good rest are vital for all people, menopausal women included. Poor sleep contributes to irritability and mood changes in the waking hours the following day when household chores and caring for grandchildren are part of the routines. Although women may cope with milder symptoms, more severe psychological symptoms would benefit from intensive counselling by experts in the field and perhaps with addition of medication like anti-depressants and drugs that reduce anxiety.

The common psychological symptoms experienced in post-menopausal women are shown in Table 4.1 below.

Table 4.1: Common psychological symptoms

1. Depression
2. Anxiety
3. Loss of memory and concentration
4. Loss of confidence
5. Unloved feelings
6. Feeling of unworthiness
7. Tiredness
8. Difficulty in making decisions

Many symptoms of the menopause mentioned above are subtle in the beginning and may be dismissed as part of aging. Others may label them a 'being nutty or neurotic'. The previous mental status prior to menopause has an effect on severity of manifestation later in life. The more a woman is stressed, the more symptomatic she becomes. In fact hot flashes are worse off in 'more stressed women'. The more informed a woman is on psychology and the menopause, the more likely she would come forward to complain of the problem. Observational studies also indicate that women from the more affluent society complain of psychological problems compared to those who are in the lower socio-economic society. This could also be due to access to health care. All physical ailments have a psychological component that needs to be addressed in treating women. The depression that follows a fracture of the hip with hospitalization is obvious. Psychological stressors present independently in the older individual even if there is little physical ailment. A third component that contributes to psychological disease is called 'the domino effect; which was alluded to above. For instance the women who is distressed because of severe and repeated episodes of hot flashes and night sweats becomes both embarrassed and irritable and would find it difficult to concentrate on her daily work. She sleeps poorly and this affects the performance the next day. She becomes more irritable and begins to have frequent mood changes that affect everybody around. Such a domino effect can be effectively reduced with treatment of the primary problem i.e hot flashes and night sweats.

Psychological Rehabilitation

Three aspects of psychological issues have been mentioned:

1. Symptoms due to physical effects of estrogen deprivation
2. 'Domino 'effect due to some disorders directly related to menopause (hot flashes etc.)
3. Defined psychological symptoms like depression, anxiety and unloved feelings

Symptoms due to estrogen deficiency are easily treated with medical hormone therapy and excellent relief is seen especially when prescribed for treatment of hot flashes, night sweats and urogenital atrophy. This supports the value of estrogen as a good hormone in indicated cases.

Patients who suffer from depression and other vague symptoms like anxiety would require a proper assessment so as to find the cause for such problems. Elaborate evaluation of the psychological state would explore past mental status and illnesses, family support and possible triggers that have added stress to the women and clues that may by interviewing the woman and also the family. A woman in the older age group is psychologically vulnerable so as to be crippled by multiple stressors that are overt and hidden.

Explorative discussions with firm constructive counselling techniques are effective and should be employed in treatment. One must not be restrictive in prescribing medication as an easy solution but facilitate the women who are severely affected by arranging for expertise in family counselling and cognitive counselling. As there is a lack of clarity about the cause of psychological symptoms in many instances a combination of counselling and medication are frequently required. Individualization of treatment is necessary for optimum results.

Treatment options

Treating psychological problems in post menopause requires skills in determining the cause as they are not due to hormone deficiency alone. Consultations should not be hurried with the wrong notion that medications alone would solve the problems. At times the family is also interviewed apart from the woman who seeks treatment. Some treatment options that are use in treating psychological problems are outlined below:

- Antidepressants—for treatment of depression, insomnia, anxiety (in some cases), hot flashes and night sweats are reduced to some extent
- Medical hormone therapy—benefit seen in mood elevation with estrogen but mostly inconclusive
- Cognitive behaviour therapy—used with anti-depressants, essential adjuvant to enable women cope with problems
- Family therapy—removes stressors and contributes to family support
- Counselling—helps solve personal and situational problems and promotes exploration of hidden views and concepts
- Meditation and 'mind over matter' are Eastern Philosophical approaches with techniques learnt from experts, can be done in groups or alone. Aim to divert wrong thoughts because of distressing situations.

Sexual Problems

Cultural hindrances and personal attitude to sex has masked the magnitude of sexual problems in many societies. The frequency of sexual intercourse in couples varies but certainly it decreases with advancing age. Sexual problems are not openly discussed and not volunteered unless enquired into during medical consultations. Many women shy away from discussing sexual problems.

More than 40-50% of women have sexual problems in the post-menopausal years. These could range from poor libido, lack of desire for penetrative sex, painful intercourse (dyspareunia) and dry vagina. Personal disability and that of the partner are factors that places sex low on the priority list.

a. Dyspareunia (painful coitus)

Painful intercourse or dyspareunia is due to the drying effect of the vaginal and other genital organs with estrogen deficiency. The cells of the vaginal lining wither and the lining atrophies making the vagina tighter (narrowing) and shorter (retraction). Attempts at intercourse are painful and difficult as the vagina also lacks lubrication. This is primary reason why sex is avoided.

Local application of estrogen cream improves the tissues of the vaginal facilitating intercourse.

Apart from atrophy of the tissues, some women may have prolapse of the uterus, bladder and rectum. The internal organs descend on straining in mild cases and remain prolapsed in severe cases making sexual intercourse both difficult and embarrassing.

b. Loss of libido

Loss of libido is a fairly common reason for avoiding coitus. This complaint may not be volunteered by women unless specifically questioned.

Two aspects of loss of libido are recognized in post-menopausal women:

i. Loss of interest in sex
ii. Loss of ability to respond to sexual stimulus

Much of the treatment for correction of loss of libido is directed to both the woman and her partner's attitude to sex. Physical disability like prolapse, vaginal dryness and atrophy, and atrophic vaginitis needs to be evaluated and corrected. Personal views on need for and resumption of coitus should be expressed so as to get suggestions and methods to improve sexual health. Open consultation with both partners is essential to explore the problem and if suggested treatment is acceptable. Addition of small amounts of male hormone TESTOSTERONE has been shown to improve libido in postmenopausal women.

CONCLUSION

The psychological aspects of menopause are varied and multifactorial. Whilst some symptoms are directly related to estrogen withdrawal with atrophy of the ovaries, others are due to changing personality and difficulty in adapting to changed environment and relationships. The vulnerable woman is prone to depressive illness and anxiety in the post-menopausal years. These need to be identified by family and practitioners as they are amenable to treatment using a combination of cognitive behavioural therapy and antidepressants. Estrogen therapy helps overcome vasomotor symptoms and atrophic vaginitis contributing to a better quality of life. Sexual problems are often not openly communicated and hence consultations should address this aspect directly. These disorders can be treated as various treatment modalities are available.

CHAPTER 5

THE HEART AND BLOOD VESSELS IN AGEING WOMEN

The heart and blood vessels are referred to as the CARDIOVASCUALR SYSTEM. The heart is intimately associated with blood vessels especially in relation to the development of high blood pressure. HEART ATTACKS refer to the sudden obstruction of the coronary blood vessels resulting in MYOCARDIAL INFARCTION. The coronary blood vessels nourish and oxygenate the tissues of the heart muscle (myocardium).

Blood vessels become stiffer as one grows older and the inner linings become damaged as a result of deposits of fat called ATHEROMA resulting in narrowing of the lumen. Narrowing of blood vessels result from atheromatous plaques and also spams of the vessel, both of which increase the pliability (resistance) of the vessel consequentially resulting in high blood pressure (hypertension)

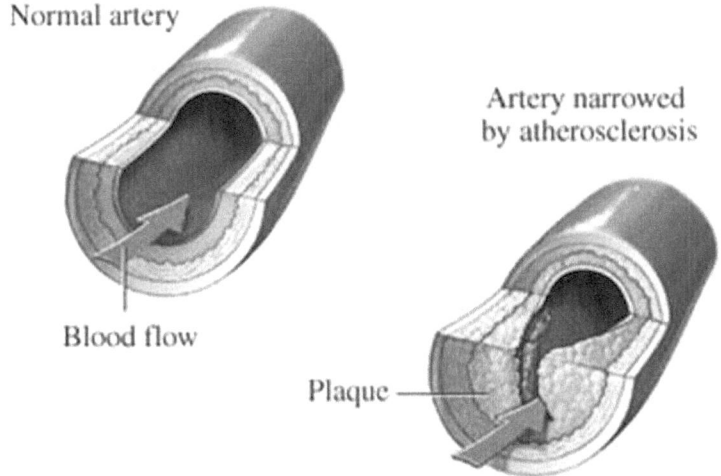

Normal artery

Artery narrowed
by atherosclerosis

Blood flow

Plaque

Fig.5.1 Atheroma in Blood Vessel

When the lumen of a coronary blood vessel is narrowed significantly due to plaques of atheroma they become narrow and do not sufficiently perfuse myocardium (muscle of the heart) resulting in myocardial infarction. Chest pains and shortness of breath are consequences of poor tissue perfusion of heart muscles. Myocardial ischemia occurs when there is diminished blood flow with narrowed lumen size, a prelude to myocardial infarction. The chain of events in coronary heart disease can be summarised based on the spasm of blood vessels and eventual decrease and complete absence of oxygenated blood to heart muscles.

The risk of heart disease in women increases with age. Heart disease is the leading cause of death in women over 40 years old, especially after menopause. Recent estimates in the United States show that over 400 000 women die of heart disease each year. The rate of coronary heart disease is about 2-3 times higher after menopause.

The myth that has been held for several decades is that hormone therapy containing estrogen reduces heart disease. Although research over several years favoured such approaches after menopause, more recent studies have not shown benefits in those with existing heart disease. In fact data shows that some forms of estrogen therapy may be harmful. The current concept is that hormone (estrogen and progestogen) is no longer recommended to postmenopausal women to protect them against heart disease.

Heart disease and gender differences

Although cardiovascular disease and death rates from this disease in woman is lower than men before menopause, data indicates that after 44 years of age, there is a similar rise in both men and women reaching equal numbers by 85 years. The chance of finding coronary heart disease in postmenopausal women aged 45-50 years is three times higher than that of women who are menstruating at the same age.

The incidence of ischemic heart disease in postmenopausal women in the United States is twice that of deaths related to osteoporosis and is much more common than breast cancer deaths. Women in the postmenopausal age will be wary of the fact that cardiovascular disease is the major cause of death in women beyond 50 years in the West.

Heart disease contributes to 45 % of all deaths in women in US. The probability of having a heart attack in the next five years is 10-20% in the presence of:

I.   Chest X-rays showing a minimum amount of calcium in women without symptoms
II. Metabolic syndrome (condition where there is obesity, diabetes mellitus, hypertension, low LDL-cholesterol and high triglyceride levels in the blood)
III. First degree relative having had heart disease (before 55 in male and <65 in female)

TABLE 5.1: Cholesterol and Lipid (Fat)

Serum Lipid Levels			
	Total Cholesterol mg/dl	LDL-Cholesterol mg/dl	Triglyceride mg/dl
Normal	<200	<130	<200
Elevated	200-240	130-159	200-499

Cholesterol has turned out to be a bad word among health freaks and the lay public. Lipids refer to all sorts of fats. They appear to be related to coronary heart disease. Elevated total cholesterol (>200mg/dl) and LDL-cholesterol (>130mg/dl) with decreased levels of HDL-cholesterol (<35mg/dl) are associated with an increased risk for cardiovascular disease (Table 5.2).

Table 5.2: Risk Factors for Cardiovascular Disease

i.	Elevated blood total cholesterol
ii.	High blood pressure
iii	Angina or previous myocardial infarction
iv	Cigarette smoking (>10 sticks a day)
v	Obesity >30% of ideal weight
vi	Lack of exercise
vii	Male sex
viii	Being East Indian
ix	Family history of premature death from heart disease (<55 years)
x	Diabetes mellitus
xi	History of stroke

Fat in our body comes in many forms, some of which are very important in metabolic processes of cells. One gram of fat would give 9 Kilocalories of energy compared to 4 Kilocalories for an equal amount of carbohydrate and protein.

Of the fats or lipids that are associated with formation of atheroma's (plaques of fat) in the blood vessels eventually leading to both coronary heart disease and stroke are CHOLESTEROL and TRIGLYCERIDES.

Cholesterol and triglycerides cannot freely float around blood without being attached to proteins called 'Apoproteins'. The entire complex in which fats are transported in the blood is called LIPOPROTEINS.

Five major lipoproteins are present in our system:

i. Chylomicrons
ii. Very low density lipoproteins (VLDL)
iii. Low density lipoproteins (LDL)
iv. High density lipoproteins (HDL)
v. Intermediate density lipoproteins (IDL) or remnants

High density lipoproteins are formed in the liver and small intestine. They play a scavenger role in removing cholesterol from tissues. They protect blood vessels from becoming clogged up with atheroma. They are good lipoproteins.

Low density lipoproteins are the product of VLDL and are considered 'bad' proteins as they are the route of atheroma formation on the inner lining of blood vessels. As cardiovascular disease becomes more prevalent in the later years following menopause, a finding thought to contribute to this increased risk is dyslipidaemia in post-menopausal women. Increases in total and low density lipoprotein (LDL) cholesterol increase with age accelerating after menopause. This is associated with decreases in high density lipoprotein (HDL) which has cardio-protective effects. These changes explain the increase in rates of coronary heart disease, myocardial infarction and stroke in post-menopausal women (Table 5.3).

Table 5.3: Three major diseases in postmenopausal women in the US	
Disease	Incidence per 100 000
Cardiovascular disease	1000
Osteoporosis	530
Breast cancer	310

Blood cholesterol can be measured using the finger prick test or from blood drawn from the veins of the arm. Normally the latter (venous blood) is preferred. A 12 hour fast overnight is advised before blood is drawn for assessment of Cholesterol and Total Lipids. It would be better for the attending physician to counsel the woman before performing the test so as to prepare oneself for correct treatment should the test results be abnormal. Many factors like age, ethnic group, cigarette smoking, gender, and family history need to be considered when the test results are interpreted for risk scoring.

Treatment

In treating patients with high lipid levels, three strategies are adopted apart from adopting a healthy life style. A doctor should be consulted for sufficient counselling in the presence of abnormal blood lipid levels.

i. Diet modification
ii. Exercise
iii. Medication

Diet Modification

Manipulating one's diet so as to offer sufficient calories with a balance of 60% carbohydrate, 20% fat and 20 % protein requires both discipline and commitment. A discussion with a dietician in order to achieve ideal weight and adhering to a meal plan especially among those with high total cholesterol is advised. Saturated fat tends to clog blood vessels and hence one should seek unsaturated fats either as mono- or polyunsaturated forms.

While polyunsaturated fat has the advantage of lowering all types of cholesterol; mono-unsaturated fat (found in olive oil) tends to reduce bad LDL cholesterol, without reducing the good HDL-cholesterol.

Food derived from plants has the advantage over animal food in having much less saturated fat. Nuts and olives contain high amounts of 'bad' fat.

Exercise

Regular and programmed exercises have been shown to lower LDL-cholesterol and triglyceride levels. Additionally, they increase HDL-cholesterol and help maintain weight. A detailed discussion appears in Chapter 8.

Other conditions like diabetes, hypertension and obesity should be optimally managed with both dietary restrictions and medication. If indicated.

Medication

If lipids levels remain high after about 3 months of diet modification and exercise, medications are advised in consultation with a doctor. Four groups medication are used to lower lipid levels. These are:

- Statins (3-hydroxy-3-methylglutaryl coenzyme A (HMG-CoA) reductive inhibitors
- Fibrates (gemfibrozil, clofibrate, and fenofibrate)
- Niacin/nicotinic acid
- Bile acid binding resins (cholesterol and cholestyramine)

The statins decrease levels of total cholesterol leading to an increased number of low-density lipoprotein (LDL) receptors, increasing catabolism of LDL and clearing LDL from the circulation. The statins are excellent in lowering LDL cholesterol may even elevate high-density lipoprotein cholesterol (HDL-C).

The fibrates reduce triglyceride synthesis and may increase very low-density lipoprotein (VLDL) levels. Niacin (Vitamin B2) lowers total cholesterol and triglycerides in high doses.

Whether a single medication or more than one is required will depend on the lipid profile. The attending doctor would advise the best option. If a woman with high lipid level is compliant to the medication, a reduction would be apparent within a month of starting medication. Blood levels of lipid profiles would be required to be done periodically to check for response.

Role of Estrogen

Historically, two landmark research studies are quoted that discussed the role of estrogen on the cardiovascular system. The Framingham Study of 1985 did not show any protective role on the heart. However, the Nurse's Health Study differed in their conclusions demonstrating the protective effect of estrogen in reducing heart disease. When the Framingham Study was re-analysed it indicated a protective effect when women between the ages of 50-59 were compared for dying or not dying of coronary heart disease.

Further, data in the 1990s showed that in women who have had their ovaries surgically removed had a higher risk of coronary heart disease. This risk apparently was reduced when estrogen therapy was initiated.

Estrogen have been said to have a positive effect on lipid levels in the body. Apart from reducing total cholesterol in the blood and low density lipoprotein, it also increases high density lipoprotein. This favourable effect of estrogen is said to be seen no matter what preparation of estrogen is administered. The WHI (The Women's Health Initiative trials) attempted to evaluate the value of estrogen alone, estrogen with progestogen in women who have an intact womb and without mediation; they were testing the effect on breast cancer, fractures and cardiovascular system. The details are best viewed in scientific journals as the statistics need to be viewed carefully and will need further explanation. In summary when both estrogen and progestogen (specifically CEE +MPA) were administered there was a 24% overall increase in coronary heart disease especially those who had higher baseline LDL cholesterol at the beginning of the study. The estrogen alone arm of the study (CEE) i.e women who did not have a uterus, aged between 50-79 years the study was stopped in 2004 ahead of schedule because of increased risk of stroke. They concluded that after 7.1 years of hormone treatment there was no cardiovascular protection overall. However, a lower risk of heart attacks was seen in those between 50-59 years. Since the results of WHI were released there have been several reports that looked at other confounding factors that need consideration in evaluating the value of hormone and other interventions. Age at entry of the study, weight of women recruited, smoking habits and alcohol has effects on the functioning of the heart and the coronary vessels. The Kroon's Early Estrogen Prevention Study (KEEPS) has been re-looking at many of the factors studied in the WHI and would help women make choices as to the way the hormones and other interventions should be used in the menopausal years.

The WHI Coronary-Artery Calcium Study (WHI-CAS) evaluated 1064 women between 50-59 years using cardiac CT and noted that estrogen alone (CEE) had a favourable effect on calcium plaque build-up in coronary vessels during the 7.1 years the women were on compared to those with no hormones (40% lower). Such information needs to be factored in when counselling women for or against use of hormones to prevent coronary vessel disease.

Conclusions

It is generally surmised that the heart and blood vessels of a woman is 'younger by 10-15 years,' year for year till she attains menopause. Circulating estrogen in the reproductive years appears to have a positive effect in protecting women from heart disease. After menopause several factors increase the chance of heart disease. These include obesity, sedentary life style, atherosclerosis and diabetes mellitus. Diet modification and exercise have moderating effects on heart function and are encouraged. Hormone therapy for reducing heart disease is not recommended.

CHAPTER 6

OSTEOPOROSIS

Two long term complications women suffer after menopause is osteoporosis and cardiovascular events like coronary heart disease and 'heart attacks'. Cardiovascular disease is discussed in Chapter 5. Osteoporosis refers to BRITTLE or FRAGILE BONES. Both men and women develop osteoporosis as they age. However, women tend to show marked thinning of their bones especially in the vertebral bone (spine), hips and wrists soon after menopause sets in, indicating that estrogen has a protective role during their reproductive years.

Apart from old age and estrogen deprivation, several other factors contribute to osteoporosis (Table 6.1). Some of these include genetic predisposition, physical activity and physical exercises, body weight, smoking and dietary habits.

Osteoporotic women are more prone to fractures. Fractures of the vertebral spine and hips are very disabling. Bony fractures in these two sites immobilize women for several weeks to months and are a major health problem. Preventive measures including complete nutrition, exercises, hormone therapy and other 'bone enhances medication' can arrest bone loss and reduce the incidence of osteoporotic fractures. It is estimated that if loss of bone is delayed by 5 years, an overall reduction of hip fractures by 50 % may be achieved.

Fig. 6.1 shows the incidence of three common fractures by age in both men and women. There are two types of bone i.e harder cortical bone and trabecular bone. Women tend to lose 15-30% cortical bone and 10-15% trabecular bone over 10 years after menopause. Subsequent bone loss occurs at a slower rate.

Vertebral spine and hip fractures are common in women although there is an increased incidence of hip (femoral neck) fractures in very elderly men. X-rays of women beyond 65 years of age, if done routinely, would reveal osteoporotic (bone thinning) changes in in two-thirds of them. Compressed or collapsed fractures of the vertebral spine lead to loss of height (Fig.6.1).

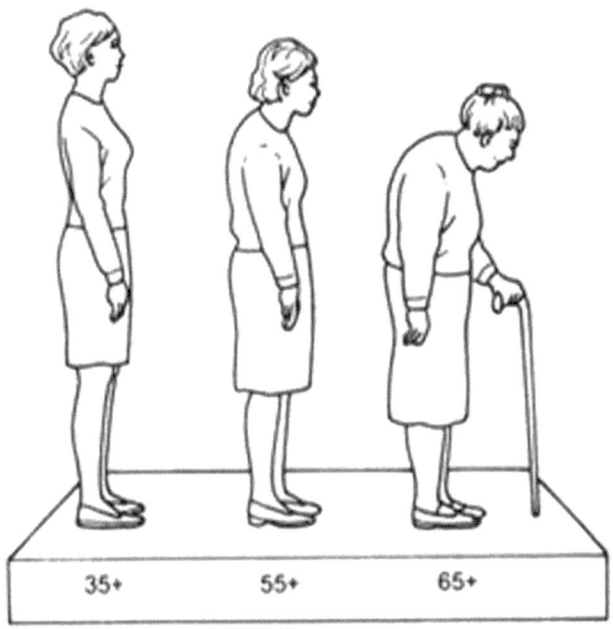

Fig. 6.1: Loss of height with ageing

THE BONE

The bone is not a static stable organ as one may think. It is a live organ which behaves like other cells in the body. Many mechanical forces act on the human bone inflicting stress injuries that warrant continuous remodelling.

Table 6.1: Risk Factors for Osteoporosis

- Female sex
- Age >70 years
- Small build
- Family history of osteoporosis
- Oriental or Caucasian
- Premature menopause <35 years
- Surgically induced menopause
- Low calcium diet
- High alcohol consumption
- Sedentary life style
- Lack of estrogen
- Long term use of steroids

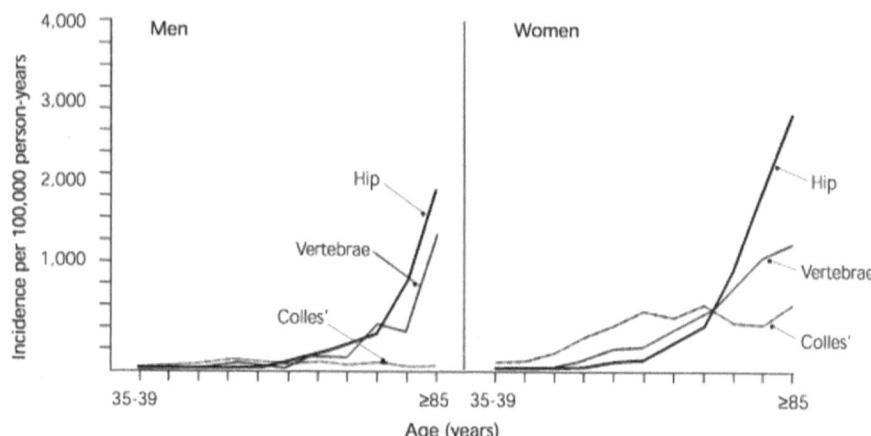

Fig.6.2 Prevalence of Fractures in Men and Women by Age
Source: Cooper C, Melton LJ 3d. Epidemiology of osteoporosis.
Trends Endocrinol Metab 1992; 3:224-9.

Peak adult bone mass or bone density is a medical term that refers to the maximum amount of bone a woman develops. Two major factors determine bone density:

i.   Genetic factors
ii. Hormonal factors.

If a woman is nutritionally deprived in her childhood and adolescence, the peak bone density would be severely affected. About 95% of peak bone density is achieved in adolescence.

i.   Remodelling of Bone

Bone is made of packets of bone cells which are closely bound together. Of the two types of bone mentioned i.e compact cortical bone and more loosely bound trabecular bone, it is the latter that is of importance in the osteoporosis process.

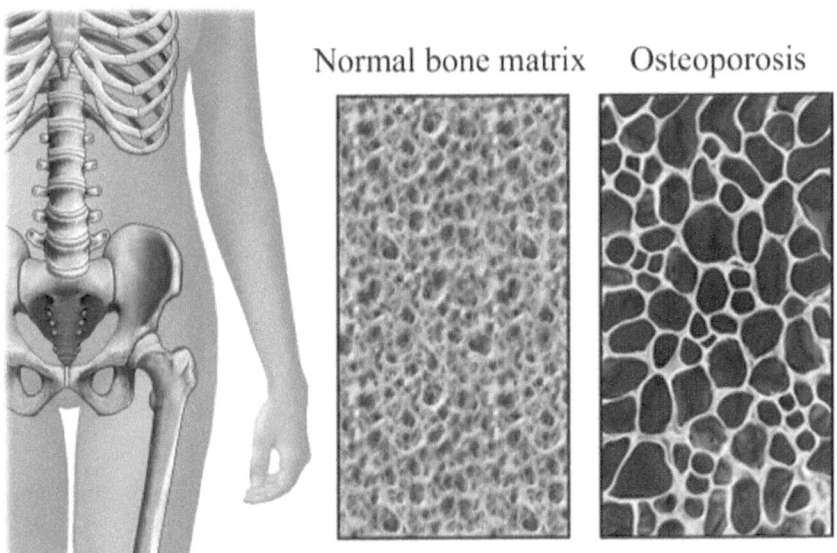

Normal bone matrix   Osteoporosis

Fig.6.3: Bone Breakdown and Remodelling

It was stated in the beginning that bone is not static. It undergoes a continuous remodelling process through the action of two types of active cells:

a.   Osteoblasts
b.   Osteoclasts

During younger years of life, activity of these cell types is coupled closely working in harmony so as to maintain an intact skeleton. A hole or a pit appears as older cells are removed. This pit gets filled up by osteoblasts.

Osteoblasts have a positive action in 'bone formation'. On the other hand, osteoclasts cause bone loss-'resorption of bone'. The harmony existing between bone formation and bone resorption is lost after menopause with the latter overtaking bone formation resulting in bone loss. It is also seen that ageing has a dampening effect on bone formation and osteoblastic function. Additionally, bone resorption is indirectly affected by Vitamin D and certain other hormones especially from the parathyroid gland. 'Excavation' of bone, however does not seem to be hindered by calcitonin.

Bone remodelling occurs at a faster rate in the young, taking about 12 weeks to complete a cycle. As one grows older, bone formation is slower taking about 16-20 weeks to complete. This could be the reason for greater loss of bone seen with ageing. The architecture of the bone also changes with age resulting in 'brittle bone' becoming detectable by the age of 30-40 years. At this age, however, there is no minimal change in bone density. However, should the patient have chronic ailments like absence of menstruation for more than 6 months (for reasons other than pregnancy), anorexia nervosa and ovarian failure, bone loss occurs at a more rapid rate?

Vulnerable areas often affected by bone loss at menopause are the vertebral spine resulting in wedge fractures and compressed fractures culminating in shortening of height, hips (neck of femur) and wrist (resulting in Colles' fractures). The loss of bone is very rapid in the first five years after menopause. Trabecular bone in the vertebral spine is lost at a rate of 1-8% per year.

ii. Vulnerable Bone Sites

Certain bone sites that have been mentioned above are more vulnerable to both bone loss and fractures after menopause (see Fig. 6.1). The vertebral bone tends to fracture following osteoporosis rather silently and may not be noticed by the woman unlike fractures of the hip and wrists. Backache and loss of height are prominent features of vertebral bone fractures.

Hip fractures involve the neck of the femur (thigh bone). They frequently occur in women past 65 years of age following accidental falls. Less than one third of women are restored to their previous functional state following treatment of hip fractures in this age group.

Table 6.2: Bone Loss (Trabecular) by Age

Age (Years) (vertebral, radius, neck of femur)	Percentage loss per year
40–49	0.5-10
50–59	3.0-5.0
>60	0.5-1.0

Falls on the outstretched hand injures wrists resulting in fractures of the end of the radius bone. Such fractures are called 'Colles' fracture'. Treatment involves applying a plaster of Paris over the hand and the lower forearm for a period of 3 weeks. Healing occurs with a deformity (appearing like the neck of a swan) as there would be some degree of displacement of the affected bone. Movement of the wrist is encouraged as soon as the plaster is removed to avoid stiffness of the wrist.

iii. **Detecting Osteoporosis**

Osteoporosis is a disease of progressive bone loss, often associated with an increased risk of fractures. The term osteoporosis literally means "porous bone." Diagnosis of osteoporosis is preferably done by measurement of bone mineral density (BMD) using X-ray energy.

Routine X-rays are usually not done to detect osteoporosis unless some disability is detected or a fall has occurred. Common modalities available for detecting osteoporosis include:

a. Plain X-rays

Plain X-Rays of the skeleton can detect fractures of bones and the presence of osteoporosis. Loss of trabecular pattern is graded (Singh index) to denote degree of osteoporosis. However, they are not sensitive enough to monitor the improvement seen with therapy.

b. Computed Tomography

To measure bone density, important bone sites need to be selected. The skeletal spine and the neck of the femur are the common sites selected for research studies in osteoporosis as they are more prone to fracture following falls in the elderly. Trabecular bone, unlike cortical bone exhibit changes related to osteoporosis. CT scan can distinguish cortical and trabecular bone distinctly and be used to monitor bone density.

With the advent of three dimensional CT scanning techniques (Quantitive CT) better images are derived and are more informative. The high radiation from CT scanning (ten times more than conventional CT scanner), however, is a limiting factor in its routine use.

c. Dual Photon Absorptiometry (DPA)

The principle behind this technique is the emission of two energies using photon beam. Two distinct energy peaks are present. One energy peak is absorbed more by the soft tissue. The other energy peak is absorbed more by bone. Bone mineral density is measured by subtracting the soft-tissue component.

d. Dual Energy X-Ray Absorptiometry (DEXA)

Dual-energy X-ray absorptiometry (DEXA) is similar to DPA, but instead of a radioactive isotope an X-ray source is used. The DEXA scanner produces two X-ray beams, each with different energy levels. One beam is high energy while the other is low energy. The aim is to measure amount of X-rays that pass through the bone for each beam. This will vary depending on the thickness of the bone. Based on the difference between the two beams, the bone density is measured. The radiation exposure from a DEXA scan is said to be very much less than when one undergoes a normal chest X-ray. The hip and the spine are commonly X-rayed and the procedure does not take more than 20 minutes.

e. Ultrasound

Ultrasound has no radiation and can be used to measure BMD. The ultrasound beam is directed at the bone selected for analysis. However, the results are not as precise as DEXA. If the bone density is detected to be low on ultrasound usually a DEXA examination will be required.

f. Peripheral Bone Density Testing

Bone mineral density (BMD) at peripheral sites e.g. the radius of the forearm, phalanges of fingers, or calcaneus (of the feet) can be measured using cheaper portable devices (Fig. 6.3). BMD assessment for the general population could be done with rapidity. The main problem is that BMD varies according to the skeletal site and low bone density in the hips and spine may be missed. In the postmenopausal woman, trabecular bone loss in the skeletal spine occurs first because of high bone turnover. It is advisable for BMD to be measured using DEXA for postmenopausal women up to 65 years.

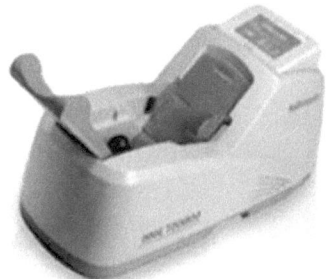

Fig. 6.4 Measuring BMD of the Foot (Snoots 3000)

Apart from measuring bone densities using the above methods (collectively called BONE DENSITOMETRY) there are, in the blood, certain substances which are produced as a result of bone remodelling. It would be the logical to measure the products of bone remodelling. However this is not commonly done in clinical practice as they cannot be used as a measure of response to medication or hormone therapy.

iv. Preventing Osteoporosis

Women suffering from disease states like disorders of the thyroid gland and parathyroid gland, rheumatoid arthritis and those on prolonged steroid therapy are prone to osteoporosis. Adequate stabilization of excessive functions of the thyroid and parathyroid glands are essential. Specific measures need to be taken to retard the onset of osteoporosis in women who suffer debilitating diseases like arthritis as many of these patients may have been on steroid therapy for prolonged periods.

The following group of patients are advised to have BMD measurement of hips and spine using DEXA:

- Medical hormone therapy or those on bone enhancing medication (bisphosphonates, selective estrogen receptor modulators
- If the woman's mother has had hip fracture
- Smoking
- Thin and tall women

- Medications associated with bone loss
- Disease associated with low bone mass (hyperthyroidism, organ transplantation, malabsorption, hyperparathyroidism, and alcoholism)
- History of previous fragility fracture

What does the Bone Density report tell us?

The bone density report will have two terms i.e T-score and Z-score. BMD correlates well with fracture risk.

T-score

The T-score is the number of standard deviations (SD) above or below that of a young adult mean BMD of a person of 20 years. When the SD is 1SD (-1) below the mean, one can assume that the woman has twice the risk of a fracture of a woman with normal BMD. This risk increases to 4 times if the T-score is (-2). Other risk factors that should be considered are age and how mobile the woman has been. This gives an idea about muscle strength and factors that could contribute to falls i.e loss of balance and falls due to poor eye sight.

Z-score

The Z-score is the number of SD the bone density measurement is above or below the value expected for the patient's age. A Z-score lower than—1.5 is suggestive of osteoporosis related to an underlying disease-disorder. Further investigations are done so as to identify the disease and treat accordingly.

Regular weight bearing exercises and weight control are central to maintaining good health in the menopausal years. This is discussed in detail in Chapter 8. Most woman often look for vitamins, food supplements and drug therapy forgetting simple daily measures that can prevent falls and strength muscles and joints. Medication to retard bone resorption and prevent early onset of osteoporosis are currently marketed.

Woman who have had their ovaries surgically removed early in life before natural menopause for medical reasons benefit from both medical hormone therapy and bone enhancing medications. Premature menopause occurs before 40 years and is candidates for medical hormone therapy to prevent osteoporosis if there are no contraindications.

Osteopenia is a precursor to osteoporosis and can be detected by measuring BMD. Gourlay et al (New England Journal of Medicine, 2012; 366:225-33) measured BMD according to T-scores on women >65 years old and followed them up for 15 years. They categorised women as normal when the T-scores was (-1) and osteopenic if T-score was (-1 to -2.5). They noted that those who were normal or had only mild osteopenia did not progress to osteoporosis till after 15 years. However, if the T-score was in the moderate or severe range, they developed osteoporosis between 1-5 years. These results would help women to decide on how frequently women should have DEXA done. Those with a T-score (-1.5) or higher would only need to have BMD determined after 15 years.

Preventing and Treating Osteoporosis

Medications have been popularly used to both prevent and treat osteoporosis for over four decades. Some medications are known to slow the rate of bone loss or increase bone thickness. It is also evident that noticeable though small amounts of new bone growth can reduce risk of fractures. Apart from taking drugs for osteoporosis, one needs to get calcium and vitamin D. A healthy diet and regular exercises are equally important. Physical activity is not only good for bone health but protects against premature deaths. A Taiwan study involving 250 000 people showed that just 15 minutes of exercise a day improved survival in both men and women (Wen et al Lancet 2011; 378:1244-53).

Common drug therapy for osteoporosis

Two classes of medications are now available. One group slows the resorption of bone reducing the rate of osteoclastic activity (most of these are listed below). The second group promotes bone formation (osteoblastic activity). These included medication like teriparatide and more recently added drug, nitroglycerin.

Bisphosphonates

These drugs are known to slow the rate of bone thinning. Bisphosphonates and strontium ranelate effectively reduce fractures in women with osteopenia. Use if these drugs for 3-5 years are recommended in osteopenic women as data shows bone resorption is slowed resulting in less fractures. Little information is available as to how long treatment should continue. Recent studies suggest that only those with established osteoporosis with T-score of below (-2) should be treated beyond 5 years when bisphosphonates are administered due to side effects *(Whitaker and Black et al, New England Journal of Medicine, 2012;366:2048-51)*.

The medications prescribed are expensive and there are side effects. Bone strength may be adversely affected by prolonged use of bisphosphonates for over 5 years. Although the numbers reported are small, one study by Park-Willie et al (JAMA 2011; 305:783-9) reported a slight increased risk of fracture.

Raloxifene (Evista)

This SERM (selective estrogen receptor modulator) slows both bone thinning and also increases bone thickness.

Calcitonin

Calcitonin is a naturally occurring hormone which regulates calcium levels and is integral to the building of bone. It tends to slow the rate of bone loss when administered as either by injection or a nasal spray. In women who have had compression fractures of the vertebral bone, pain relief would be seen calcitonin injections.

Parathyroid hormone (Forteol)

This hormone has to be given by injections to postmenopausal women who are at an increased risk of fractures. Another medication which has a similar effect is Denosumab.

Calcium and Vitamin D

Calcium is often taken as a food supplement in both young and old. A majority of women get sufficient calcium and vitamin D from normal diet and sunlight. There is much hype about food supplementation in the ageing population.

A report from the USA (Slomski, JAMA 2011;305:453-6) found that 5 % of women over 50 years of age in USA were consuming calcium above the upper limit for safety. This would put them at a risk of kidney stones and even cardiovascular disease. Supplements of calcium and vitamin D are only required when there is inadequate intake of vitamin D and calcium.

Daily calcium required is 1200mg and about 800 I.U. vitamin D. Going outdoors and exposure to the sun for 15 minutes twice a week would be enough to meet vitamin D requirements.

A study by Bishoff-Ferrari et al (NEJM 2012; 367:40-9) involving 35000 subjects concluded that high dose supplementation was somewhat 'favourable' in preventing hip fractures. However, the United States Preventive Task Force (Kuehn, JAMA 2012; 306:225-6) states that 'supplementation with low dose vitamin D and calcium was not effective in prevention of fractures in postmenopausal women' when 400 IU vitamin D and 1 gram calcium was administered.

These studies translate to saying that supplements should be given only to women who do not receive adequate dietary calcium. There is a real risk of developing stones in the kidney in those taking supplements for 7 years even with low doses of calcium.

Should one determine blood levels of vitamin D before initiating treatment? This test is very expensive. Any proposal to determine blood levels of vitamin D would open the doors for unnecessary testing and is generally discouraged.

Hormone Therapy

Women who had had hysterectomy (womb removal) and have menopausal symptoms benefit from short courses of estrogen for 1-2 years. The hormone is also effective in preventing osteoporosis. Current opinions vary in using hormone therapy for osteoporosis especially for periods longer than 5 years. There is a need to discuss long term hormone therapy with your attending doctor. In women who have an intact uterus (i.e not surgically removed) and require medical hormone therapy should be prescribed a combination of estrogen and progesterone to avoid tumours growing in the endometrium (lining of the uterus).

Nitroglycerine

This cheap and readily available medication has anti-osteoporotic effects apart from causing the coronary blood vessels to dilate and reduce workload on the heart. Although more research is needed, it may become a useful medication to prevent osteoporosis. Jamal et al (JAMA 2011;305:800-7) studied the effect of rubbing 15 mg of the 'rub-on gel' of Nitroglycerine nightly for 2 years and found 7% increase in cortical bone thickness of the thigh bone (neck of femur bone mass density).

Conclusion

Osteoporosis is a well-defined process of ageing and is considered a silent disease. Once menopause sets in the protective role estrogen in maintaining skeletal bone ceases with rapid bone resorption making it brittle and prone to fractures. The backbone (vertebral spine), hips and wrists are frequently involved in osteoporotic fractures in menopausal women. By the age of 75, 25% of women would have suffered vertebral fractures, 15% a hip fracture and another 15%, a fracture of the wrist.

Prevention of osteoporosis should begin in adolescence with adequate dietary calcium and physical activity so as to attain peak bone mass.

Estrogen therapy reduces the incidence of fractures if it is started early in menopause. However, current views are that long term estrogen use is not appropriate for prevention of osteoporosis when risk-benefit ratios are considered and that specific bone enhancing medications are currently available. These alternative medications that retard bone thinning and promotes bone thickening are preferred as they do not have the long term risks of estrogen therapy.

In patients with established osteoporosis, calcium supplement does not appear to be beneficial unless calcium in the daily diet is less than 500mg. Calcitonin may be an alternative.

CHAPTER 7

CALCIUM: MYTHS AND NEED FOR SUPPLEMENT

Vitamins and nutritional supplements have become increasing popular with retail pharmacist and supermarkets stacking a variety of tablets and gels. One such supplement is calcium. Bone needs to be fortified with calcium and vitamin D before bone loss occurs. Rapid decline in bone strength occurs by 40 years of age and this is accelerated after menopause. A discussion on osteoporosis in Chapter 6 touched on calcium needs in menopause. Much of this is also related to risk of osteoporosis. This chapter will highlight some of the facts one needs to know about calcium after menopause.

Role of Calcium in Bone

Calcium content in the adult woman amounts to about 1 kilogram. Bone mass and bone density are at its peak as the female approaches late adolescence. Bone becomes well mineralized as this stage of life. This fact should drive home the point that for maximum benefit in later life, adequate amounts of calcium should have been consumed with her diet.

Calcium requirements increase during pregnancy and while a woman is breastfeeding. If the does not take adequate calcium during these periods she may not be able to provided enough to the growing foetus and baby.

There will be no need to take calcium as a separate supplement if a woman takes adequate amounts in calcium contained in her diet. Generally a woman needs about 800-1200 gm. of calcium a day. If the dietary calcium is less than 800 mg then she should be advised to take calcium supplements. This principle would apply to older woman after the menopause where food intake may vary with physical disability, lack of exposure to the sun and inability to take a well-balanced diet.

The metabolism of calcium is rather complicated for a detailed discussion here. This mineral is required in the proper functioning of various cellular mechanisms. There must be adequate amounts of calcium in the fluids surrounding the cells of the body for efficient cellular metabolism. Should there be inadequate calcium because not enough is taken by way of diet or inadequate amounts are absorbed from the intestine, calcium stored in the bones will be mobilized to replenish the calcium of extracellular fluids.

Calcium is also lost from the body through the skin, urine and from the gut daily as part of the normal body activities. About 200-300 mg of calcium is lost each day in an adult woman who is not pregnant. If these losses are not replaced by adequate dietary calcium, calcium will be drawn from the stores in bones which inevitably contribute to increased loss of bone mass and bone strength!

Calcium lost in the urine is usually under some degree of control depending on the metabolic state of the woman. The normal kidney is capable of retaining calcium when it is necessary. On the other hand, calcium contained in diet is handled differently in the intestines. As food passes through the gut, only about 25-35% calcium is absorbed, the being passed in stools. Absorption in the intestine may be affected by problems related to digestion and its disorders. Women vary in their ability to absorb calcium. Based on absorption efficiency research in adult women, taking into consideration obligatory losses mentioned above (through urine, stools, skin) a daily intake of 1000-1200 mg calcium is sufficient.

i.   Can calcium supplements support bone mass?

In order to answer this question we need to revisit the mechanisms involved in bone resorption and bone formation. Estrogen appears to play a pivotal role in adolescence and early adult life in maintaining bone. The maximum bone mass reached in puberty and adolescence is rapidly lost with estrogen deprivation seen after menopause. Between puberty and menopause the decline in estrogen in the presence of risk factors mentioned sets the stage for the development of osteoporosis and fractures. Estrogen appears to be the major player and not calcium. Hence, prescribing large amounts of calcium supplements cannot revert the loss of bone. For instance woman who suffer from a psychological state called anorexia nervosa have prolonged periods of amenorrhoea (absence of menstrual cycles) due to estrogen suppression. These patients are prone to loss of bone which requires hormonal therapy and not calcium supplements.

When calcium levels in the blood are measured in most women, no remarkable change is seen because of the shift if calcium from bone into the blood. When estrogen and calcium are taken together, both appear to play a complementary bone—protective role. This dual action on bone metabolism maintains bone mass at its maximum, clearly, estrogen deprivation at menopause leads to osteoporosis and consequent risk of fractures.

ii. What are the other effects of estrogen?

Apart from having a positive effect on bone, estrogen appears to play an equally important role in its ability to conserve calcium in the kidneys in improving the efficiency of absorbing calcium from the intestines. Unfortunately this effective role of estrogen no longer operates after menopause. If a woman is taking adequate dietary calcium her calcium levels would not be markedly affected. Calcium supplements should be prescribed to only those women who do not take adequate amount of calcium in their daily diet.

iii. What are the common sources of calcium?

A list of calcium-rich food should be provided to women so as to educate them about how much calcium is available in various food products. Dairy products are by far the best sources of calcium. Milk, yogurt, cheese and ice cream are common foodstuff with calcium. Women concerned about fat content of whole-milk may opt for low fat milk. Yogurt products usually have low fat. Both yogurt and low fat milk are good sources of proteins and riboflavin, apart from calcium.

Other foodstuff containing calcium is dark leafy vegetables, soya bean curds and certain fish like salmon and sardines.

Calcium supplements in the form of 'pills' are available in a variety of proprietary forms. One must be careful with formulations. While some products are well established as regards to calcium content and absorption properties in the intestine, others may not be absorbed efficiently and be passed out in stools.

Foods and juices are now available fortified with calcium. Women unable to take dairy products may find such food pleasing and palatable.

Conclusion

Calcium is an important mineral for cellular functions and is vital for bone mass. Adequate amounts of calcium needs to be taken during childhood and adolescence so as to fortify bone mass and maintain calcium balance in the body. Calcium containing food is encouraged rather than calcium supplements. Estrogen appears to play a pivotal role in bone formation and bone maintenance. A woman consuming a balanced diet needs to take additional calcium.

CHAPTER 8

EASING INTO THE MENOPUASE WITH EXCERCISES

The American Council on Exercise agrees that exercise improves the quality of life and contributes to healthier life. A regular program of physical activity not only helps reduce symptoms of menopause but has a positive impact on heart disease and osteoporosis. One tends to look at exercises as being strenuous and tiring. This wrong notion is adopted by viewing videos by health freaks and magazines that promote such programmed activities that would lead to building muscle bulk. There are now professional fitness and aerobics instructors who can plan a gentler program to suit the older person. Other exercises becoming popular are yoga and Tai Chi.

No exercise program can fit all age groups and body frame. Exercise needs to be tailored to one's physical state and capabilities. Flimsy advice like 'walk more and get your weight down' is probably less helpful. Menopausal women may have medical problems like heart disease, arthritis of the knees and visual impairment. Advice for women with medical disease and physical disability would be different than for those who don't have any disabling disease.

Inactivity and leading a sedentary life are detrimental and could lead to obesity. It also leads to boredom and is not good for blood circulation. Although gardening and housework are encouraged some women would need bone strengthening exercises which are programmed for maximum benefit. Prolonged periods of bed rest leads to loss of muscle strength and even pressure sores especially following paralytic stroke. Smoking contributes to increase in cardiovascular disease, lung complications and risk of dying. Obesity and smoking has been shown to be associated with higher risk of dying (Boggs et al NEJM 2011; 363:901-08). Smokers need to give up the habit early. Current evidence shows that support group, effective counselling techniques and use of nicotine-receptor blocking agents (West et al. NEJM 2011; 365:1193-200) can help quit smoking.

Giving the Heart a Chance

Although heart attacks are uncommon during the reproductive years, the incidence equals that of men soon after the menopause after the protective effects of estrogen declines. The long held view that women's estrogen protects them against cardiovascular disease has been contested by new views expressed by Vaidya et al (British Medical Journal, BMJ 2011; 343:d5170). Women with long standing hypertension and diabetes mellitus are at a higher risk of coronary heart disease. Obesity and a lack of exercise increase the risk of heart attacks.

Coronary heart disease is due to plaque of fat called thrombus forming on the inner lining of the blood vessels supplying the muscles of the heart. Regular exercise and weight reduction improves blood circulation and is protective against coronary heart disease. In the unfortunate event a woman suffers a heart attack, apart from specific treatment of the disease, exercise would be advised, so called cardiac rehabilitation programme.

i. Prevention is better than cure

The old adage 'prevention is better than cure 'is appropriate at this stage of life. Changes in lifestyle, refraining from smoking and leading an active life including regular exercise are vital in preventing heart attacks. Improvement in blood circulation would be achieved by actively increasing the heart beat above the resting heart rate of about 72 beats per minute. Try locating the pulse in the wrist (radial pulse) by placing three fingers along the vessel lying lateral to the tendons of the wrist. It would be sited at about 2 cm below the thumb over the wrist. Count the rate of the pulse for a full minute to determine the rate. In more athletic women the rate may be slower than 72 beats per minute. As one begins her exercise like brisk walking or running, the demand for oxygen increases leading to the heart pumping at a faster rate. This is reflected in an equal increase in the radial pulse rate.

It is true that with low intensity workout, you won't be able to enjoy the benefits of exercise. But, strenuous exercises may raise your pulse rate beyond limit. Intensive exercises, performed with very high heart rate do not give you any extra benefit. In fact, such exercises can damage the heart muscle. So, you are supposed to calculate the target heart rate during exercise and work within the range.

Table 8: 1 Pulse rate (minutes per second)

Adult	72-80
Pregnancy	85-90
Exercise	90-120
Well-conditioned athlete	40-60
Age adjusted maximum heart rate for women	(226-age) =?

The pulse rate of younger women would be lower than menopausal women. Age and weight affect resting pulse rate with the overweight woman have a higher pulse rate. Menopausal women who have health problems and obesity should seek consultation before beginning an exercise program. The mathematically minded 50 year lady, in the absence of disabling heart and lung disease, could increase her heart rate to a maximum of 176 beats per minute (FORMULA: 226-50= 176) while exercising. This target could be achieved slowly over a period so as to acclimatize oneself to such a rapid heart rate. To begin with she should perform moderate exercise aiming to increase the heart rate 65% (i.e 82 beats per minute). With continued regular work ups this could be increased to a tolerable rate, say 85% of 126 i.e. about 110 beats per minute. Eventually she could go the maximum rate depending on her tolerance and capability. However, these figures are arbitrary and women wanting to take on exhausting exercise should seek professional advice.

There are many instructional manuals available for those inclined towards formal structured exercises. Many find it more fun when they do exercises in groups. Clubhouse and gyms are good places to go to where a bit of socialization can take place apart from fulfilling the objectives set in improving muscle and bone strength through exercise programs. The cheapest form of exercise is of course walking and bicycling. Many parks in housing estates have walking paths together with sites for biometric exercise. Walking briskly so as to increase the heart rate to the desired rate can be achieved quite easily with constant practice. Walking or slow jogging should be sustained for a period of 30-45 minutes.

Warming up prior to partaking is any form of exercise is recommended. This gets you into gear and loosens up the muscles and joints. A warm down period is equally necessary after brisk walks or jogging. A busy individual should engage in whichever exercise that suits her for at least about 3-4 times a week.

Benefits of Exercise

The benefits of exercise are numerous. One of the known benefits is delaying bone loss and sustaining bone density. A study in Boston involving 239 women aged between 43-72 years who were not on estrogen therapy but walked for more than 7.5 miles per week had high bone density than those who walked less than a mile per week. In the same study the researchers found that walking slowed down rate of bone loss from the lower limbs, confirming that walking is a beneficial form of physical activity as far as bone is concerned.

Jochanan Stessman and colleagues evaluated the benefits of exercising for older adults by recruiting 1862 individuals (Archives of Internal Medicine 2009; 169(16):1476-1483) and concluded that physical activity improved both functional status and longevity. Age of participants ranged from 70-85 years. In their study, anyone who did less than four hours of activity per week fell under 'sedentary' and those who performed vigorous physical activity like jogging or swimming at least twice a week over 4 hours or walking daily at least for an hour were 'physically active'.

The benefits related with physical activity were observed not only in those who maintained an existing level of physical activity, but also in those who began exercising between ages 70 and 85. The authors write: "Although the mechanism of the survival benefit is most likely multifactorial, one important finding was the sustained protective effect of physical activity against functional decline. Physical activity may postpone the spiral of decline that begins with inability to perform daily activities and continues through illness and death. Exercise improves cardiovascular fitness, slows loss of muscle mass, reduces fat, improves immunity and suppresses inflammation."

A bonus of regular exercise apart from improving muscle strength, heart and lung function is a positive effect on both depression and decline in cognitive function. Those women who are disabled should try to do some form of exercise within their limitation assisted by carers. A program for muscle strengthening is essential and this is done with the help of experts and recommendation based on initial assessment of each person. The more able older person could work up their capacity for the additional benefits mentioned moving to more intense activities.

Source for information on exercise for the older person:

http://www.who.int/dietphysicalactivity/factsheet_olderadults/en/index.html

ii. Muscle mass, fat and metabolism

It is inevitable for one to lose muscle mass as one ages and this leads to decreased metabolism. This is because muscles tend to 'burn' more calories than fat. It is said that one can lose about one kilogram a year through this process if we don't preserve muscles through weight training and exercise. Weight gain develops with a lack of adjustment of the number of calories we consume in tandem with the drop in metabolism after menopause. Of course the genetic makeup of a woman would also influence weight gain.

iii. Types of exercise

We have discussed two types of exercise; one is walking briskly and working up in a gymnasium. As long as the benefits of the exercise are known, it does not matter what form of exercise one does. There are underlying scientific principles that clearly show the benefits of exercise in menopausal women.

Swimming is an excellent exercise for all ages. If this is the preferred form, it is perfectly alright as long as it is regularly done and an increase of heart rate is noted. Swimming, however, is not a weight bearing exercise.

Jogging is a popular in the younger age group. As one grows older they may find jogging strenuous. In the menopausal age be mindful of the surface one runs as balance needs to be maintained to avoid falls. Cycling is a useful alternative and can be increased in intensity according to one's capability and tolerance. Games like tennis and badminton are competitive in nature but could still be enjoyable. Ballroom dancing is coming back to fashion and appears to be popular among certain groups of people. Golfing is another popular game but the pace may not be fast enough to increase heart rate it is taking through slowly.

Table 8.2: Loss of calories during common physical activities (based on 65 Kg woman)

Activity	Speed (mph)	Calories/hour
Walking	2	240
Cycling	6	240
Swimming	25 yard/min	275
Jogging	5.5	740

Table 8.3: Benefits of physical activity for older adults (World Health Organization)

Lower mortality (all causes)
Lower rates of : • Coronary heart disease • High blood pressure • Stroke • Type 2 Diabetes Mellitus • Colon cancer
Higher Level of: • Cardiorespiratory and muscular fitness • Healthier body mass and composition • Improvement in sleep pattern • Feeling of wellness due to ENDORPHIN release
Improved blood biochemistry that prevents diabetes mellitus and enhances bone health
Higher functional level: • Lower risk of falling • Cognition • Mobility

Conclusion

Apart from maintaining a trim body, exercise has innumerable benefits in the menopausal women. Domestic work may not be adequate to derive the suggested benefits. It can be summarily stated that exercise that lasts for about 30 minutes, 3-5 times a week, and that which raises the heart rate above the resting levels has huge benefits. Age should not be factor in getting involved in physical activity, neither should diabetes and hypertension. Exercise keeps the heart strong and improves the pumping function, lowers blood pressure, regulates blood sugar and firms up muscles. It has positive effects on controlling blood cholesterol and above all maintains a healthy body and mind.

CHAPTER 9

NUTRITION IN MENOPAUSE

Food and diet are two terms that of often not well understood as distinct entities. The consumption of food is essential for growth and repair of body tissues. As one grows older the type of food consumed changes due to changing needs, wants and dislikes. Food is used to please, treat, celebrate, reward and even manipulate situations. Eating patterns and social circumstances affect one's food intake. Age related diseases like diabetes and hypertension will require a change in food contents with particular attention being paid to calorific and salt intake. Both calorific value of daily food intake and contents as to its variety will become vital in ensuring a balanced diet is taken It would be rewarding to know a little about food contents and be aware of eating patterns as these can be manipulated to our advantage in the golden years.

Diet is often misinterpreted to be aligned to reducing fat and containing high fibre food or special meals. Diet is a way of eating of eating and should be approached in that manner.

i. Attitudes and approaches

It is not uncommon to see weight increase with increasing age. Weight excess and obesity is a worldwide problem not only in older persons but in the younger population too. Why is this? This is largely due to consuming more food than is required resulting in more calorie intake compared to what is lost. Excess calories are converted in the body to be stored as fat. Fat deposition is often disproportionate with a large part being stored in the waist. Increasing weight puts a strain on the heart as the heart has to work harder to keep the circulation going to nourish the tissues of the body. Further strain is also put on the knees and the spine.

As one grows older there is a change in body image and probably self-esteem. A higher food intake is seen to be consumed when a person is depressed. A sedentary life with lack of exercise is not uncommon. With changed home circumstances, children moving out to pursue their own careers the 'empty nest syndrome' can contribute to both psychological issues and diet changes. Children moved out to pursue their own careers leaving mum lonely! Does it matter if I am a little fat? My husband does not mind the way I look anyway! These are some of the thoughts that may grow through a woman's mind in the older age. Some women who are already overweight do not know or are capable of changing their dietary habits to attain ideal body weight.

ii. Balanced diet

Starving and skipping meals are not effective means of losing weight. A good balanced diet should consist of the following:

- Carbohydrates 60% (may be changed to 40-50% depending on body type)
- Proteins 20%
- Fat 20%
- Micronutrients of vitamins and trace elements
- Fibre
- Minerals and water

It is not adequate to be aware of the percentage of the constituents if we are not sure as to how much of each component to consume. The huge amount of information on the internet and lay press send mixed messages of what is good and what is bad. There is a huge industry out there that promotes a variety of food products that is claimed to be good for the body. A combination of a lack of good information and ill advice are pushing people to purchase these nutrition products that have filled up the shelves of pharmacies and supermarkets.

The number of calories required per day depends on body habitus and the type of work one does. To achieve an ideal body weight one needs to factor in several other issues. Certain medical disorders one suffers from require one to be selective in food choices. A dietician could assist drawing a meal plan to achieve the ideal weight especially for those with a medical problem. Suppose a person weighs 80 Kg and the ideal weight is calculated to be 60 Kg based on body frame, taking into account height, weight and age, there is an excess of 20 Kg to be shed. Then calories are calculated so as to maintain a balanced diet and at the same time, aim to lose the excess weight. Here again there is a need for understanding the principles if calculation, the reasons why shedding excess weight is essential and a huge amount of motivation required, as to how this can be achieved.

For a fairly active female, the daily calorie requirements will vary from 25-30 calories /Kg. If one wishes to achieve a weight of 60 Kg instead of 80 Kg, then the total body requirements are:

$$60 \text{ Kg} \times 30 = 1800 \text{ kilocalories}$$

Should heavy work be involved the woman would require additional calories and this has to be added to the formula. An obese woman who is expected to lose excess fat is advised a lower amount of perhaps 20 calories / Kg and not 30 as suggested above.

Considering that the 60 Kg woman above who needs about 1800 kilocalories per day, the food or meal plan would then be worked out so that she would get about 60% of it as carbohydrates i.e 1080 kilocalories. She will need another 360 kilocalories as proteins (20%) and 360 kilocalories as fat (20%).

Now this is easy arithmetic, but how do we translate this into our daily food intake?

This would be based on knowledge of how many calories each gram of the elements mentioned.

Carbohydrate	1 gm = 4 kilocalories
Protein	1 gm = 4 kilocalories
Fat	1 gm = 9 kilocalories

You would notice that 1 gm fat has more than double the calories found in carbohydrate and protein. Using this information, one can then translate calorie requirements into grams of food. Dieticians would provide the actual amount of food types that would meet the requirements of calories per day.

In the above example 1080 calories of carbohydrates will translate to 270 gm food containing carbohydrates. One should work out the weight of fat and protein in a similar way.

Labels on food packages in most countries will have contents of food together with measurements and conversions to calories printed onto food cover. It will be helpful to get the services of a dietician so that local food measures and daily requirements may be easily worked out.

Fruits and raw food in their natural state are a good source of fibre, energy, vitamins and minerals. Processed food is inferior to fruits and raw food as they contain permitted preservatives, colouring, sugar and added salt. Sundried fruits like raisins are superior to that found in cans which have excess sugar.

Green vegetables contain essential minerals and vitamins. Preparation of vegetables is important to preserve the ingredients. Stir fried and blanched food retains vitamins than prolonged cooking and mashing vegetables in hot temperature.

Pre-packed food is inferior to fresh foodstuff like fresh fish and meat. If you are meat eater, be aware of the different types of meat that is being selected. White meat and chicken are superior to red meat of beef and mutton.

A reasonable amount of water needs to be consumed if we life in a tropical climate where the room temperature can rise up to 35 degrees Celsius. Water consumption is preferably timed between meals and not during meals. Herbal tea and fruit juices are good especially if they are fresh. Be mindful that readily available fruit juices that we get from the shelves have added sugar and preservatives and add on to total calories. Strong coffee and tea have caffeine and can affect sleep patterns. If vasomotor symptoms are present it is advisable to avoid caffeine.

Table 9.1 Healthy Eating Habits

1. Do not overeat
2. Avoid excessive salt
3. Avoid fried food
4. Trim visible fat from meat prior to consumption
5. Eat more white meat and fish
6. Increase fibre in diet
7. Grill good rather than fry

Eating Habits

We talked about eating patterns and eating habits. Try to keep meals simple. Tell others of your plan so that you can adhere to your meal plan rather than be cajoled into eating what you would normally avoid. Some women have the habit of deferring dinner till late night. Remember that there is a lot of work that needs to be done by body metabolism and heart. Food has to be digested and converted into small bits to enter the blood circulation from the intestines. This takes time. Have dinner early so that there is enough time for digestion. Go for a short walk after dinner. Otherwise indigestion and sleep disturbances may occur.

Food should be chewed slowly and thoroughly so as to facilitate digestion. Try to partially fill the stomach rather than overeat. Meals should be taken regularly and according to one's appetite. Wisdom, motivation, adequate exercise and good eating habits will guide the older woman to attain ideal body weight.

High Fibre

Adding adequate amounts of leafy vegetables and eating wholemeal bread as opposed to white bread are both healthy and ensures adequate amount of fibres in our diet. High fibre is not absorbed from the intestine easily adding bulk to stools, contributing to good bowel movements.

Oat bran has made waves in many communities compared to wheat products. It is considered soluble fibre. Although there are controversies about its good effects, apparently its 'soluble fibre status' permits to draw cholesterol from bile reducing blood cholesterol levels. If oat bran is not readily available Quaker Oats including the 'instant' variety is recommended as a substitute for normal breakfast cereal. Rice bran is said to have similar effect as oat bran.

Fat and Cholesterol

We dealt with 'bad' LDL-Cholesterol and animal fat in Chapter 5. The subject has been well dealt with in many health articles.

What more is to be known about fat and cholesterol? Fast food products, canned cooked meat and sausages contain high amounts of fat. Deep fried meals, pastries, curry puffs have high calorie and fat content contributing to increased calories and need to be considered in working daily calorie requirements. All salad dressings have high calories due to oil and fat content.

Food preparation and selection of food can help reduce fat content. White meat is preferred to red meat. Even when preparing white meat like chicken, it healthy to remove the skin and visible fat. Should there be a craving for thick gravy or 'fast food fried chicken' limit it to alternate weeks so that consumption is reduced markedly. Butter is avoided but his should translate to using thick layers of margarine on bread!

The limitation in fat and cholesterol should begin early in life. It not only prevents excess fat deposition but also prevents development of atherosclerosis and high blood pressure.

Salt Restriction

Daily salt intake is recommended by the American Guidelines (2010) to be less than 1500 mg per day). Salt intake is reduced in patients with high blood pressure. Salt retains fluids and is not good for high blood pressure. In preparing food, one should be cautious in the use of savoury sauces and 'aji-no-moto'. Oyster sauce, tomato sauce and barbecue sauce should all be restricted. Highly processed food which contains added salt, like salted fish, is bad for one who has been advised to restrict salt for medical reasons. Above all, avoid making salt and readily sauce available at the dining table!

Vitamins and Minerals

There is much hype in promoting vitamins and various food supplements in improving health. Many retail outlets run huge promotions round the year claiming how various products improve general health, prevent medical disease and promote memory. Numerous vitamin preparations are readily available including herbal preparations.

Most vitamins and minerals are available in foodstuff consumed daily. We only need tiny quantities of vitamins and trace elements and most are readily available in balanced food. Food preference and food preparations may affect availability of some vitamins. If green leafy vegetables are over cooked, vitamins and essential food elements may be denatured.

If a particular vitamin deficiency is present, then specific vitamin supplements must be given. It must also be remembered that food preference and medical ailments would change food consumed and can affect vitamins needs. Diabetes mellitus is associated with deficiency of certain types of vitamin B. Some intestinal disorders are linked to inability of the gut to absorb essential food elements. If the women are unable to chew because of dental problems this can affect food consumption indirectly causing deficiency is both calories and quality of food.

One vitamin that may become deficient as we age is vitamin B12 which is found in animal proteins like poultry, eggs, milk fish and fortified cereals. We need a daily intake of 2.4 micrograms daily of B12, a vitamin that plays a role in maintaining healthy brain and spinal cord levels. Memory and cognitive functions are affected in vitamin B 12 deficiencies. It is also known that less acid is produced in the gut as we age and acidity is required for proteins to release B12 after ingesting animal proteins.

High homocysteine levels are allied to decline in cognitive function and dementia. One vitamin that can prevent this is folic acid. Folic acid is prescribed to pre-pregnant women to prevent development of neural tube defects in the foetus. It appears to be equally important that adults continue to take folic acid. Folic acid is also known to have anticancer properties and its relationship to homocysteine indicates it would also reduce coronary heart disease. A dose of 400-600 micrograms daily is recommended.

In chapter 7 calcium was discussed. Trace elements like iron, magnesium, fluoride, magnesium etc. are all necessary for effective cellular function and should be present in food consumed daily. Iron taken as supplements, causes the stools to be 'dark' and may cause some women to be constipated. Calcitonin is needed for prevention of osteoporosis. Fluoride increases trabecular bone and should be included in our diet.

Large doses of vitamin D or its derivative calcitriol has not been proven to be great value in improving bone mass. Women who are aged and have poor dietary intake are the ones who should be prescribed recommended amounts of vitamin D. Because of promotional efforts by retailers, many women seek recommendations as to which vitamin and food supplement are good for them. They feel better, at least psychologically, when they take certain food supplements. Adequate counselling should be given and each woman needs to be evaluated as to the need for adding food supplements and vitamins to their daily intake. A balanced diet provides most trace elements and vitamins for daily requirements in healthy women. If at all food supplements and vitamins are required women need to know the cost-benefit of such additional supplements. Remember that vitamins and trace elements are needed in very tiny amounts daily.

Vitamin E is an essential vitamin for improving the metabolic function of cells. It value was prominently discussed in the 1990s as a wonder drug in the menopause together with vitamin C, promoting both as effective anti-oxidant. Even claims in improvement of cardiac function were reported after cardiac by-pass surgery. 'Free radicals' caught the eye of both scientists and doctors as the 'culprit' that affected cellular function and there was a drive to look for agents that would negate the bad effects of 'free radicals'. Both vitamin E and vitamin C came into the picture. Vitamin E was reported to 'scavenge' fat soluble 'free radicals' while vitamin C was supposed to clear water soluble free radicals. Vitamin C is found in citrus fruits, vegetables, broccoli, asparagus and vitamin E is found in nuts, seeds and oil.

Labels on all food stuff that is packed have a list of the ingredients and we have to look at the contents of vitamins and food supplements contained in it. Organ meat contains most trace elements we need. Green leafy vegetables have adequate iron supplements. Spinach, carrot and cabbage contain beta-carotene which is a vital substrate for precursor of vitamin A. β-carotene has beneficial effect on blood vessels and appears to have a protective effect against cancer.

Daily requirements of vitamin A are found in a variety of foodstuff including liver and eggs. Women need 2300 I.U. Vitamin A daily. Vitamin A promotes bone growth and good vision and appears to be essential for maintaining a good immune system. The Carotene and Retinol Efficacy Trial, a lung prevention trial was stopped before its scheduled completion because of an increase in cancer. The Institute of Medicine (US) does not recommend vitamin A supplements to the general population.

Fish derived omega-3 fatty acids have been reported to have numerous health benefits. Salmon, tuna and trout are good sources of omega-3 fatty acid. They appear to have anti-aging properties and have benefits in reducing stroke, heart disease and Alzheimer's disease. Many of these claims have not been well established in scientific studies and more work needs to be done before recommendations may be made. A nutritionist and your general practitioner need to be consulted.

Current opinion on use of nutrients including vitamins cautions on over-dosing oneself with such supplements. Large doses of vitamin D are known to cause nausea, diarrhoea and even damage the kidney, if consumed over a long period. Excess vitamin A may lead to osteoporosis. It makes sense that unless a person has deficiency of a particular vitamin or trace element, there is little benefit in consuming additional nutrition supplements. Women who feel it necessary to take nutritional supplements and herbal products must be given adequate information to make decisions wisely. Most vitamins and trace elements can be derived from a balanced diet. Professional advice on food supplements, vitamins and various trace elements would be cost-effective and could avoid adverse side effects. The Dietary Guidelines of America reiterate that vitamin and mineral supplements are 'not a replacement for a healthy diet'. Many of the recommended vitamins and trace elements are found in naturally occurring food and we should encourage a balanced diet rather than recommending additional supplements.

Table 9.2. Recommended Daily Allowance of Vitamins and Minerals (EU)

Vitamins	RDA	Minerals	RDA
Vitamin A	800 µg	Calcium	800mg
Vitamin D	5 µg	Magnesium	375 mg
Vitamin E	12 mg α-TE	Iron	14 mg
Vitamin K	75 µg	Copper	1 mg
Vitamin B1	1.1 mg	Iodine	150 µg
Vitamin B2	1.4 mg	Zinc	10 mg
Niacin	16 mg	Manganese	2 mg
Pantothenic acid	6 mg	Potassium	2000 mg
Vitamin B6	1.4 mg	Selenium	55 µg
Folic acid	200 µg	Chromium	40 µg
Vitamin B12	2.5 µg	Molybdenum	50 µg
Biotin	50 µg	Fluoride	3.5 mg
Vitamin C	80 mg	Chloride	800 mg
		Phosphorus	700 mg

Source: http://www.nhs.uk/news/2011/05May/Documents/BtH_supplements.pdf

Supplements that are used for treating ailments

Glucosamine sulphate has been widely used by women who have joint pain especially osteoarthritis of the knees. The scientific evidence is not strong enough to conclude that it is effective in reducing pain. There are reports that minimal pain relief is obtained in some. Again women should be given enough information to make choices in using glucosamine sulphate. Women going for surgery should cease taking glucosamine for at least two weeks.

Ginseng is another herbal preparation that has been reported to improve memory and cognitive function. Again there is a need to wait for more conclusive evidence for recommendation. Currently it does not appear to reduce dementia and cognitive decline. Side effects like high blood pressure have been reported. Hence a medical consultation is advised. Evidence is also inconclusive in the use if Gingko in its benefits in improving memory and reducing dementia.

Taking zinc supplements as soon as one gets a cold appears to reduce the duration of cold. In fact, taking zinc supplements regularly appears to reduce cold attacks. Only recommended doses of zinc from reputed manufacturers should be consumed as there are side effects like metallic taste, nausea, abdominal pain and diarrhoea. There is no conclusive evidence that taking high doses of vitamin C reduces risk of getting cold. Rise in blood sugar is seen in people with diabetes mellitus consuming vitamin C. Reputed scientific reviews (Cochrane Review) on use of high doses of vitamin did not show prevention of infections. Echinacea, an herbal product, also does not help in reducing attacks of cold.

MyPlate for Older Adults

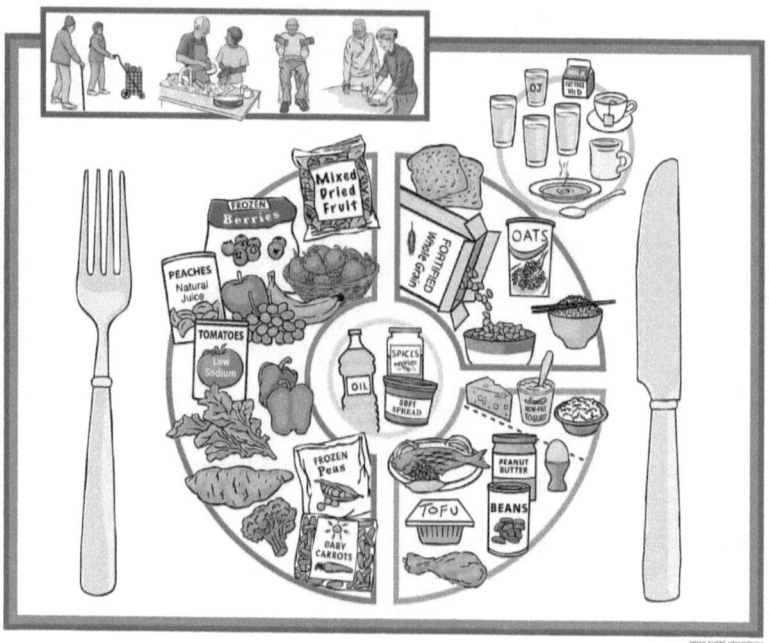

Fig. 9.1. Food Pyramid for older people
Source: http://nutrition.tufts.edu/research/myplate-older-adults

Saying 'no'

Most people are courteous and we entertain though food and drinks. Feasting is part of communal celebration and social eating is part of life. In Asian countries the numerous festivals that are celebrated inevitably ends with feasting. Inviting friend and family over for a meal is part of socialization. Food outlets promote feasting by making food available throughout the day. Many a time we consume food because of circumstances and to act 'civil'!

Table 9.3 Body Mass Index

Body Mass Index	Kg./M^2
Healthy weight	18.5-24.9
Overweight	25.0-29.9
Obese	>30

When we are on a meal plan we need to curtail the desire to consume food as it is presented. This can be very difficult but we would require additional motivation and commitment to say 'no' when we are presented with food that is not suitable for you. Though it may be impolite to refuse to attend a function, it is not impolite to decline a dish if the reasons stated are clear to both parties. Soft drinks and syrup drinks are a huge source of calories because of the amount of sugar it contains. These should be omitted from the meal plan. Snacking on high calorie-containing food like white chocolate and ice-cream between meals should be a no, no. Ceasing to eat when we feel that our stomachs are half or three-quarter full is a good strategy. Do not wait for the satiety centre to signal you to stop. Over-eating just because food is readily available is certainly a clear way to gaining excess weight.

Obesity is a major health problem worldwide and needs to be addressed so as to prevent and reduce complications of diseases like hypertension, diabetes, mellitus and coronary heart disease. When the BMI (see Table 9.3) exceeds 30 Kg/M2 there must be serious attempts to get into a weight reduction programme.

Boggs ET at (New England Journal of Medicine, 2011; 365:901-8) researched on 34 000 black women in the US over 15 years relating their risk of dying to the body mass index (BMI). The lowest death rate was seen in those with a BMI between 20-24 Kg/M^2 and this rate doubled at a BMI of 40 Kg/m^2. A similar trend was seen in those of European descent and the main cause of death was cardiovascular disease.

Buffet-style food at restaurants and major food outlets is of major concern to many of us as they promote excess food intake at all ages. It is not uncommon to see people queuing for food and filling their plates to the full of each and every item displayed. There must be a clear plan as to what is to be consumed so that one can adhere to the meal plan that has been drawn to derive from the benefits of healthy eating. It is good practice to survey the food display area and be able to select only food that fits your 'calorie-budget'.

The Tufts' University Nutrition Scientists popularised a modified food pyramid for older people above 70 years and this was later replaced by the Myplate for Older People (Fig. 9.1). This contains a colourful arrangement of food that is preferably consumed. Although total calories decline with aging, the nutritional requirements remain fairly constant. Included in the diagram are three activities that contribute to good health i.e physical activity (walking and resistance training) and light cleaning. The Myplate program also emphasises the need to take adequate fluid so as not be dehydrated. Frequent coffee and tea consumption leads to a decline in thirst in older folks.

Conclusion

A balanced diet with sufficient calories for one's age and body frame will achieve ideal body weight. Increases in weight as we grow older, puts a severe strain on heart, lungs and joints. Bodily functions are affected and both diabetes and hypertension are more difficult to manage if ideal body weight is not maintained. Due attention to healthy food habits and a food culture need to be in place in families and friends to assist older people to adhere to an established meal plan. A healthy nutritional status promotes good health and reduces complications of chronic disease present in older people. People may purchase nutrient supplements provided they have been sufficient information on the benefits and alternatives so as to make their own choices. They should also be cautioned on the adverse effects of such supplements. The older woman should access current information from authoritative and regulatory bodies like the National Health System (NHS document on supplements, 2011) and FDA (USA) before consuming 'over the counter 'nutrient supplements.

Reference

1. Buhr G, Bales CW. Nutritional supplements for older adults: review and recommendations. J Nutr Elder 2010: 29(1): 42-71.doi:10.1080/01/01639360903586464
2. www.nhs.uk/news/2011/05May/Documents/BtH_supplements.pdf
3. The Department of Health set Dietary Reference Values (DRVs) for the UK population (in 1991).
4. NHS Choices: www.nhs.uk
5. Bjelakovic G, Nikolova D, Gluud LL, Simonetti RG, Gluud C. Antioxidant supplements for prevention of mortality in healthy participants and patients with various diseases. Cochrane Database of

Systematic Reviews 2008, Issue 2. (http://onlinelibrary.wiley.com/o/cochrane/clsysrev/articles/CD007176/abstract.html)

6. USDA National Nutrient Database at http://ndb.nal.usda.gov/ndb/search/list.

7. http://hnrca.tufts.edu/publications/tufts-nutrition-magazine/

CHAPTER 10

TAKING CONTROL OF YOURSELF THROUGH REST AND RELAXATION

Menopause is an inevitable biological event that affects women as they approach 50-52 years. There is abundant literature on the supposed effects of menopause on tissue and body function. When we discuss the plethora of events around the onset of menopause, they do not appear to be directly associated with the physiological effects of endocrine changes alone but also to changed outlook of life and personal relationships. A multitude of psychological problems manifest around the menopause that include mood swings and sleep disturbances.

Women at this age of life may play multiple roles—homemaker, career women at the height of their professional practice, politician and grandmother. Several stress factors are operational that would impact on intrinsic bodily functions that may be wrongly ascribed to hormonal deficiency. Consultation with a physician would permit evaluation and exploration of the issues presented and also an opportunity to assess attitude and personality of the individual so as to suggest correctable measures which include techniques in taking control of one through non-pharmacological methods. Learning to know oneself and how to cope with stress are essential for adaptation to changed circumstances of life.

Psychological 'defence mechanisms' need to be developed to overcome the effects of stressful situations. In most instances, the family and spouse need to come into the picture to reinforce these defence mechanisms. Family support means family awareness and this goes a long way in assisting menopausal women to live a quality life after the menopause.

The value of taking rest

What is meant by rest? Does it mean getting enough sleep? Women are often 'busy-bees'. If they are at home, they are always doing things around the house even if they are career women. They are cleaning the house, changing the curtains, dusting the furniture as they grumble over the maid's performance. They worry about what to cook and also how the share market is doing. The stresses on woman, as they grow older, are even more especially if the children are not progressing well academically and if they have to nurse an ill relative at home. Imagine a woman who is approaching 50 and has three adolescent children and an executive husband who is out of the house early and returns only at night. What if she holds a part time job and has no house help except for the maid who comes in the weekends to clean the house and the bathrooms. Imagine if this lady also has her 70 year-old widower father-in law who has early stage Alzheimer's disease. The busy schedule that this lady has to keep apart from spending quality time with her children and husband when they are home would have drawn a huge amount of both energy and mental strength. All these set in motion a series of events which impacts on the psychological and physical wellness of the affected person. If the coping mechanisms are poor, depression and psychosomatic problems may ensue.

The three 'R's of rest are relax, refresh and recover strength. Asking someone to take adequate rest is easy advice but may be difficult to accomplish especially if the woman is tied up with household chores and has to mind old folks at home. Family and social support may be warranted in such instances. Family counselling may assist in adapting to the situation and getting additional help to overcome the effects of psychological stress.

a. How much sleep do we need?

There is no magic figure how much sleep a person needs. Whatever sleep a woman gets must be quality sleep that would address the three 'R's. The National Sleep Foundation of the US have developed a guide on how much sleep people need at various stages of their development. The woman in her menopause may not need as much sleep as a younger person; perhaps 6-7 hours may be sufficient at night. Disturbed sleep and family stressors contributes to both mental and physical exhaustion. Depressive feelings is a common accompanying symptom

Table 10.1: Duration of Sleep required for various Age Groups

Age	Sleep Needs (hours)
Newborn (0-2 months)	12-18
Infants (3-11 months)	15-15
Toddler (1-3 years)	12-14
Pre-schooler (3-5 years)	11-13
School-age (5-10 years)	10-11
Teens (10-17 years)	8.5-9.25
Adults	7-9

Source: National Sleep Foundation

A feeling of loneliness and not being loved can affect personality, eating habits and sleep. Depressed people have difficulty falling asleep and waken in the early part of the morning. Getting up several times at night to urinate due to urinary problems markedly disturbs sleep patterns and gives a lousy feeling the next day.

In order to get quality sleep we need to address the issue of stressors affecting sleep. Some of these stressors have been mentioned. One needs to establish a sleep pattern, a schedule one follows even during weekends and holidays. A conducive environment, devoid of noise with privacy, is essential apart from having a comfortable mattress and pillow. It has been said that taking a warm bath an hour before bedtime and avoiding caffeine before bedtime are helpful. Meals should be taken a good 3 hours before bedtime. Remember to establish consistent sleep and wake schedules, even on weekends. Regular exercises improve sleep.

Sleeping pills are not recommended on a routine basis for women with sleep pattern disturbance. Women who have poor sleep pattern need proper evaluation by physicians before medication is prescribed. Tranquillizers like Dormicum or Xanax may be necessary in a few to relief anxiety, if evident. Apart from getting a reasonable number of hours of sleep at night, short 'shut eyes' in the mid-afternoon appears to energize some old people assisting them to cope with evening exercises and activities.

b. Tackling Depression

The common question is 'Are psychological states of anxiety and depression intrinsic to menopause?' Clearly the answer is much more complex than that. Women who approach menopause appear to have 2-2.5

higher chance of developing depressive symptoms. This may not entirely be due to hormonal changes. Consider the influence of gender; far more women have depression than men, age for age. Tearfulness and irritability may manifest because of inability to adapt to changed home circumstances and personal expectations leading to mood swings. Woman who have suffered premenstrual syndrome are at a higher risk of depression.

Some of the possible factors that contribute to depressive and anxiety states have been mentioned above (stressors of life). Altered self-image and ageing are also factors that need to be considered. Increasing anxiety with palpitations and shortness of breath may be felt by some to the extent they feel panicky (panic attacks). Difficulty in remembering and a lack of concentration can be frustrating and affect normal functioning. Poor relationship with children and spouse leads to family crisis and need to be addressed as it may trigger the onset of major depressive illness.

Depression is not uncommon after the onset of menopause. In fact depressive illness is one of the most widespread ailments in old age. There may be an association of anxiety with depression in women who suffer from intolerable hot flashes and night sweats. Some relief is seen with alleviation of depressive symptoms with successful treatment of hot flashes.

Drug treatment for depressive illness should not be resorted to till proper evaluation of the complaints is done. Sympathetic handling of the affected person by a professional is advised. Both psychotherapy and family counselling may be required.

i. Elements of Psychotherapy

Psychotherapy is psychological counselling that requires the woman to engage with a psychologist or doctor trained in this field. Several sessions would be required where issues and problems will be talked through to determine the cause of depressive illness and exploring if the person can come to terms with the situation. She will be taught how to cope with unhealthy thoughts and experiences. One needs to be pragmatic by putting realistic goals for life and not be bitter if things don't go the way it is going. The aim is to learn new and alternative methods that would turn things around so that they are no longer 'stressors'. Positive thinking, adaptive methods and adjusting to crisis would improve the state of the mind and avoid feeling despondent. Cognitive psychotherapy is one form where we try to replace negative thoughts and behaviours with positive ones which are healthier and would derive a sense of pleasure. The aim is to change our own thoughts rather than try to change the situation.

Family counselling requires bringing in other members of the family so as to improve interpersonal relationships so as to develop a non-hostile environment. It is another key treatment for depressive illness. Psychotherapy is a general term for a way of treating depression by talking about your condition and related issues with a mental health provider. Psychotherapy is also known as therapy, talk therapy, counselling or psychosocial therapy.

ii. Common drugs used for depressive illness

Early intervention with psychotherapy and medication is required if depressive illness is present. Drugs are prescribed to help overcome anxiety and depressive symptoms. If depressive illness is very severe especially when suicidal thoughts are present, urgent medical attention is required.

The common drugs used are listed below in Table 10.2. A doctor's prescription is needed and close follow up is required.

Table 10.2 Common medication for depression

Group of Antidepressant	Common Medication	How they work
Selective serotonin reuptake inhibitors (SSRI)	fluoxetine (Prozac), paroxetine (Paxil), sertraline (Zoloft), citalopram	Antidepressant Few side effects May have decreased sexual desire Some have restlessness, headache and insomnia
Serotonin and norepinephrine reuptake inhibitors (SNRIs). These medications include).	Duloxetine (Cymbalta), venlafaxine (Effexor XR) and desvenlafaxine (Pristiq	SSRIs. Side effects like SSRI Can cause increased sweating, dry mouth, fast heart rate and constipation.
Norepinephrine and dopamine reuptake inhibitors (NDRIs) fall into this category. It's one of the few antidepressants that don't cause sexual side effects. At high doses, bupropion may increase your risk of having seizures.	Bupropion (Wellbutrin)	Antidepressant Can increase seizures (high dose) No effect on sexual desire
Monoamine oxidase inhibitors (MAOIs)	Tranylcypromine (Parnate) and phenelzine (Nardil Selegiline (Emsam) (patch)	Not first choice medication Food restrictions include cheese, pickles, wine, decongestants

Other medications may be prescribed apart from antidepressants depending on the symptoms. These could be to treat anxiety symptoms and to stabilize the mood. As a woman grows older she may be on other prescriptive medication for age related diseases. She should discuss about interaction of antidepressants with other medication. She should also be aware of the side effects of all drugs. Dizziness could result in falls and bone fracture.

c. Urinary symptoms and Night sweats

Night sweats are due to vasomotor instability. This involves a re-setting of the temperature centre in the brain to a higher level probably due to the release of substances like serotonin. Hot flashes accompanied by profuse sweating and night sweats can literally soak one's clothes and cause a great deal of annoyance disturbing sleep. Estrogen therapy relieves these symptoms and is the best treatment option.

With estrogen deprivation after menopause, the organs in the pelvis suffer by becoming 'shrivelled 'and small. The bladder shrinks in size and so does the urethra resulting in increased frequency of urination because of a smaller bladder capacity. Some may develop an overactive bladder where the muscles are rather sensitive and begin to contract ever so often. Menopausal women are more prone to urinary infection. All these changes occurring in the urinary system makes the woman go the toilet often, both during the day and night. Urinary infections are treatable with medication.

d. Relaxation

Rest and relaxation come hand in hand. Relaxation is not equated to LAZINESS. It relates to freeing oneself from stress and unwinding oneself. Your husband is screaming as he rushes to work ; he can't find the car key, your old father is trotting out to get the newspaper, nearly falling down as the dog rushes past him to the doorway as your son has left the front door open as he rushed off to school!. You are getting the breakfast ready in time for the kids to grab some food and the washing machine does not start! The hectic schedule mum has increases her stress levels. Although the body and mind are capable of tremendous tolerance and exertion, it will be met with fatigue, tiredness and mental agony. A variety of bodily effects result as tension builds up over the days and years. The muscles become tense and irritability and headaches persist in a stressed woman. Some stress sharpens one's senses and mind but too much of it is detrimental.

i. *Stress and Relax Response*

Stress is related to the 'Flight and Fright Response'. Much of this is under the influence of the autonomic nervous system (ANS). The two opposing systems keep the ANS functioning to keep the body going—i.e the sympathetic and parasympathetic systems. Both systems are not directly under the person's direct control and tend to work 'automatically'. So when the heart rate is too fast under the influence of the sympathetic system, it is slowed to maintain the normal rate of about 72 beats a minute through the parasympathetic system.

Interestingly, the ANS influences several vital centres in the brain. The blood pressure and heart rate are under the influence of the ANS and so are the metabolism of all cells and blood flow to tissues. Muscle tension and breathing pattern and rate are also under the influence of the ANS. When anxiety sets in as a result of some stressful event, the heart rate races up and breathing is more rapid. The muscles tense up and there may be sweating. These are all due to the release of chemical transmitters in the blood in response to stress, the 'flight and fright response'—a natural response to encounter potentially harmful events and stress. Panic attacks are an exaggeration of these responses. However, if we have adequate coping mechanisms, we would see the effect of the parasympathetic response which has the opposite effect of all that is mentioned above and calm and quiet sets in. Relaxation techniques work on self-control and how we could reduce the ill effects of stressors.

ii. *Relaxation*

Now we have some idea about the role of the autonomic system. Apart from that the cerebral cortex of the brain has specialized functions. In a right handed person the left cerebral hemisphere is dominant. May of our abilities like language, speech, questions, mathematical calculations, analytical and logical thinking reside in the left hemisphere. On the other hand, abstract imaginative thinking and creativity functions operate in the right hemisphere. Other softer skills related to emotional appreciation and feelings are equally important functions of the brain that leads to how one handles stress. So the cerebral hemispheres contribute to a large part of higher order functions. If an electroencephalogram (EEG) is done to look at wave patterns of the brain, various types of waves will be seen indicating different activities the brain does. Deep relaxation is associated with alpha and theta waves. Meditation, creativity and emotional stability are linked to these wave patterns.

Relaxation techniques should lead to relaxation of both the body and mind. Relaxation techniques operate in trying to harness strategies to take control of abnormal brain function, that which gives rise to ugly thoughts and emotional instability. Having knowledge of brain functions would enable us to use suggestions and techniques to induce appropriate thinking lessening the effects of stress.

Table 10: 3 Waves of the Electroencephalogram (EEG)

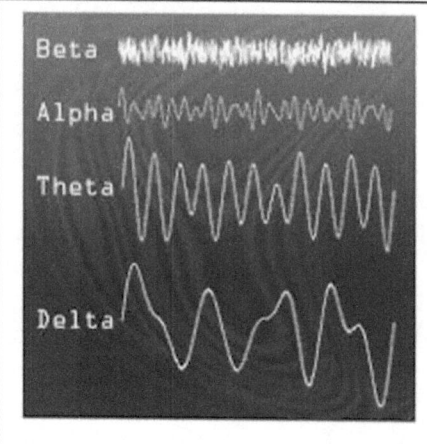	**Beta waves** Emitted when alert, agitated, tense or afraid (13 to 60 pulses per second) **Alpha waves** Emitted in physical and mental relaxation in conscious state (7 to 13 pulses per second) **Theta waves** Reduced consciousness (4 to 7 pulses per second) **Delta waves** Unconsciousness, deep sleep (0.1 and 4 cycles per second

Reference: Lagopoulos et al. Increased Theta and Alpha EEG Activity during nondirective meditation. *The Journal of Alternative and Complementary Medicine, 2009; 15 (11): 1187 DOI: 10.1089/acm.2009.0113*

iii. Meditation and Tranquillity

The dominance of the left side of the brain over the right side (in a right handed person) is related to specific functions. Each side of the brain appears to have specific functions and peak independently. During deep relaxation and meditation, however, both sides work in synchrony as they peak together. This contributes to greater mind power and self-control. Neuroscience researchers have mapped out areas of the brain that contributes to the positive effect meditation has in relieving stress and sustaining tranquillity.

Table 10:4 Basis of Relaxation Techniques

Relaxation Techniques	Basis of Technique
Autogenic training:	Uses both visual imagery and body awareness to move a person into a deep state of relaxation
Breathing techniques	Becoming conscious of own breathing.
Progressive muscle relaxation:	Involves slowly tensing and then releasing each muscle group individually
Progressive muscle relaxation	Slow tensing and then releasing each muscle group individually beginning with the muscles in the toes and finishing with those in the head.

Simple methods used

Meditation and relaxation techniques have helped people relax and unwind. A positive approach needs to be adopted so as to accept these techniques and use them on a regular basis. A state of wellbeing is realized in people who regularly resort to meditation. It is said that a conducive internal environment is created and this has a positive effect in relieving stress, healing and enhancement of the immune system. It appears to improve the physical state and overcome mental tension.

Before beginning these relaxation techniques one needs to allocate dedicated time for the practice. A state of total wakefulness is required and cannot be replaced by sleep. A quiet place is preferred so as to avoid being disturbed. Wear loose fitting clothes and assume a comfortable position. It is not necessary to squat if this is not comfortable. You need not cross your legs if you are sitting, if this not possible in view of arthritis. It is perfectly alright if you choose to lie down on the floor. The position assumed should allow good blood circulation.

Focus on a distant object. If this is not possible, close your eyes and focus on a point on the forehead. Alternatively, you could think of a serene spot or a peaceful scene; water flowing gently downs a stream. Once this is achieved, concentrate for several minutes and experience a state of relaxation. With regular practice and concentration, one can feel the relaxed and pleasurable feelings derived from the exercise.

Other techniques

- ## The Rhythm Method

Normal breathing is an involuntary process. In this technique one needs to be aware of breathing so as to have a 'control' over it. With a conscious effort you should be able to distinguish the short gap experienced between INSPIRATION (breathing-in) and EXPIRATION (breathe-out).

Begin by taking in a deep breath, pulling in the tummy at the same time. The chest muscles are held up holding it for a while. Begin counting slowly. Then breathe out, again slowly noticing the chest dropping. Become limp and relaxed during this phase.

This process is repeated several times. Ensure a period of relaxation follows each expiration.

Another rhythmic method is to focus on both thought processes and breathing technique simultaneously. Prompting yourself to relax as you take this breathing exercise assists further in successful relaxation.

As described above, you may start in the sitting position in a quiet room. You may want to keep your hands together, palm against palms with eyes closed (optional). The idea is to withdraw from any distractions from the outside world.

Take note of feelings you have, whether comfortable or uncomfortable. Be aware of the thoughts that run through your mind at this point. Follow these thoughts and then then try to keep them away for a while.

Continue the breathing technique mentioned above and learn to let go of these thoughts. Continue to say to yourself that you are now relaxing. Pay particular attention to 'RELAX' so that the uncomfortable and not so pleasant thoughts disappear.

Now learn to relax physically. You feel heaviness in your forehead and eyelids. Focus on your forehead and eyelids. Now learn to let go and relax. Feel the tension leaving the eyelids and forehead. Feel the muscles of the face, chin and jaws going lax. Feel the total relaxation of the face and head. The jaws now drop and are relaxed. Now relax the muscles of the neck, throat, chest and abdomen working you down the body. Reach the muscles of the backbone and feel it relaxed. You should feel the limpness descending down the abdomen and deep within. Then work down to relax the muscles of the buttocks and lower limbs-thighs and legs and then the feet. Let them go limp and feel how relaxed they are. Your whole body should now feel relaxed.

The technique leading to this relaxed feel can be reinforced and deepened by looking upwards with the eyes closed as if the eyes are directed above the eyebrows.

As you do this, you also begin to appreciate the deep breathing that is going on. At first they may have been shallow, but now, they are deep, and breathing is clearly in and out. You can distinguish the gap between breathing in and breathing out. The breathing is clearly a part of you!

There is an INSPIRATION and EXPIRATION phase during breathing. Learn to associate the inspiration phase with the backbone near the buttocks to the top of the head. As you breathe out, direct your attention from the top of the head to the spine. The expiration phase should now be longer. It is associated with relaxation and unwinding-concentrate on 'letting go' with expiration. Also focus on the short gaps between inspiration and expiration-relax during this intervening period. Soon two distinct phases are apparent with a relaxation phase in between. Learn to prompt this 'relax' as you breathe out and keep it longer as you repeat the process.

You will feel relaxed as you continue these techniques. The rhythmic pattern of inspiration and expiration need to be recognized to benefit from this technique. Complete the whole process over several minutes and rejoice with the relaxation you derive from it. This would be like re-charging your batteries. Keep doing these breathing exercises as a routine and rope in other members of the family.

As you contemplate as to when you are going to do the next exercise, rub your palms together and give yourself a good stretch. Release the hands and open your eyes now. For maximum benefit, the practice needs to be done on a regular basis.

- **Tension-relaxation method**

You could do this by lying flat on the floor on a mat or mattress. The aim is to learn to run the relaxation feeling from the top of the head, down the entire body to the tips of the toes. Aim to focus on certain parts of the body in the process.

Begin by tightening the muscles of the left lower limb. You can fan out the toes; push your heels away, tightening the calf, thigh and buttock muscles on the left. Draw your tummy in tightly keeping all affected muscles tight and contracted to a point of discomfort. At this point, you should keep the rest of the body muscles relaxed. Also keep the back muscles and face soft and limp. Learn this technique of maintaining one part of the body under tension which keeping the rest of the body relaxed. When you are able to do this you are performing DISSOCIATION. You have learnt to dissociate the tensed part of your body from the relaxed parts. The process is a conscious effort. Now, just breathe in, tightening the left side a little bit more. You, can then, with a slight sigh, release all the tension built up in the affected muscles from abdomen, left buttocks and thighs, calf and feet. Feel it relaxing as you let go of the tension you had built up. You can say 'relax' softly as you feel the muscles going soft.

Now repeat the exercise on the right side dissociating the rest of the body. In a similar fashion, move on the rest of the body including the upper limbs, head and neck.

Many other techniques are practiced by various groups of people including imagery, distraction, biofeedback and hypnosis. You are advised to learn methods under the guidance of experts if you feel working by yourself are not sufficient. Group therapy appears to be beneficial to some as the social interaction that goes with group practice pushes you along in the right direction. Regular practice is required to obtain best benefits.

Yoga has been practiced for centuries in India and has been effective in promoting both health and reducing stress. Basic yoga can be learnt from videos. For advanced yoga, a trainer should be consulted.

Resources

www.gpcare.org

http://www.bbc.co.uk/health/emotional_health/mental_health/coping_relaxation.shtml

Conclusion

Advising the menopausal woman to get adequate rest and relaxation is not sufficient as situations and circumstances that remain as stress factors can be depressing. The effects of menopause like hot flashes and night sweats can be both embarrassing and a cause of great discomfort. Short courses of estrogen or alternative medication are indicated in these instances. Most urinary symptoms are treatable and would improve quality of life. Personal and family counselling may be necessary in some instances. Should depressive illness be diagnosed definitive medication and various forms of psychotherapy may be required.

Estrogen therapy and lubricants are useful in genital atrophy that makes sexual intercourse painful. Antibiotics are effective in treating urinary tract infections which are common after the menopause. Should urinary incontinence and bladder over-activity be present, these are to be treated so as to improve substantially, the quality of life.

Relaxation techniques are useful to stress and certainly are worthwhile learning. Regular meditation and relaxation exercises overcome stress and contribute to maintaining sense of relieve wellbeing. Weight bearing exercises also strengthens muscles and bones.

CHAPTER 11

HORMONE THERAPIES

Hormone therapy for symptoms related to menopause has been in vogue for decades and has been beneficial in improving women with debilitating effects of hot flashes and dry vagina. Estrogen has been shown to prevent osteoporosis and improves the texture of skin. Traditionally the sex hormones produced in the body are:

- Estrogen
- Progesterone
- Androgens (testosterone and DHES)

All three types of hormones are STEROIDS and are derived from a common biochemical substrate (see Fig.11.2). Subtle differences in the biochemical formula produce hormones that have unique effects on different tissues. Certain enzymes in the body tissues are capable of transforming one hormone to another. This complex biochemical changes are beyond the scope of this book. Suffice to note that estrogen may be transformed to produce ANDROGENS in fat cells (adipose tissue). Androgens are found in small quantities in women but excess amounts would disturb normal menstrual cycle pattern.

Estrogen and progestogen (synthetic progesterone) are central to hormone therapy in menopause. Estrogen and progesterone are equally important in maintaining menstrual cycles by their coordinated effect on the tissues of the endometrium of the uterus. When the fine balance in the release of these hormones is lost disturbances in menstrual cycle pattern are evident. Progesterone and androgens play modulating roles on the effects of estrogen on tissues of the uterus, breast and hypothalamus of the brain.

ESTROGENS

Three sub-types of estrogen in the body are:

- Oestradiol
- Oestrone
- Oestriol

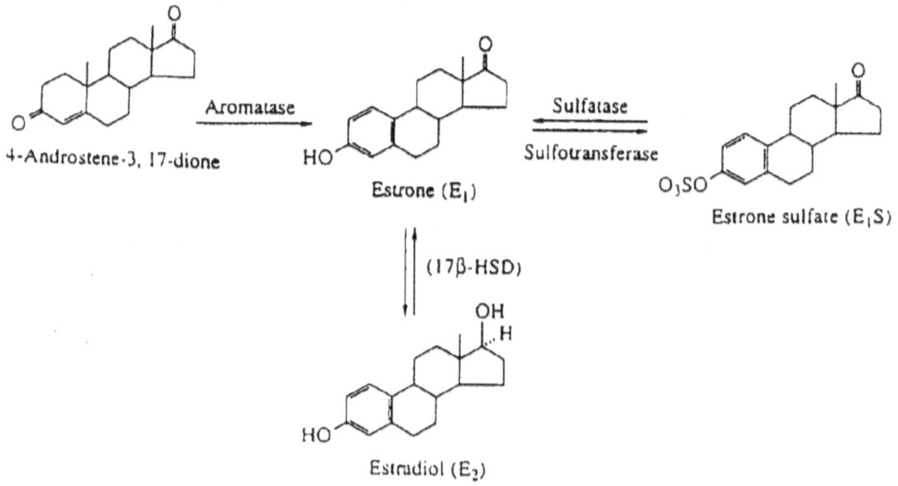

Biosynthesis of estrogens

Fig. 11.1: Chemical Structure of Steroid Hormones
Foot note: Note the similarities and differences in the chemical structure of various steroid hormones, both naturally occurring and synthetic

Estrogen is the primary hormone that declines rapidly as a woman ages. A certain type of estrogen named 17 β-Oestradiol, is of primary importance and is demonstrated to be very low after menopause. 17 β-Oestradiol levels range between 40-400 pg/dl during a 28 day menstrual cycle peaking at the time of ovulation. Following menopause this levels falls to about 30-40 pg/dl in the blood. If all the symptoms of menopause are ascribed to a decline in oestradiol, a simplistic solution to alleviate the troubling symptoms of menopause would be to prescribe oestradiol so as to overcome the deficiency of the hormone!

Prescriptive drugs containing 17—oestradiol are available for use in menopausal women. Medications available come in fixed doses. Research in this field has mandated prescription of minimum doses of estrogen for an individual depending on both effectiveness and safety. Individual differences arise because of:

i.   Variable drug absorption by the body
ii. Actual amount of drug reaching the tissues after absorption
iii. Varying compliance to medication

The issue of compliance or adherence to medication important. Up to 30% of women are known not to adhere to prescription advice for various reasons including inadequate information. Other reasons for not adhering to medication regime are side effects and fear of adverse effects like cancer and deep vein thrombosis. While significant progress has been made in the evaluation and treatment of climacteric symptoms, successful use of hormone therapy can only be achieved through education and a clear understanding of the value of hormone therapy.

PRESCRIBING ESTROGENS

Any kind of medication or drug prescribed to a person should be acceptable. Ideally it should be easily accessible, preferably cheap, and easy to consume and not cause unacceptable side effects. It is almost impossible to have such an ideal drug. Most hormone preparations are tolerated by women. Some of the side-effects mentioned are unpredictable and may be unacceptable. Unfortunately there are also undesired effects with unforeseen metabolic effects. Appropriate counselling on both need for adherence to prescription regimes and possible or known side effects assist women in their understanding of purpose of hormone therapy and also improves compliance to therapy.

As far as estrogen is concerned, a variety of drug preparations are available. Women prescribed specific preparations of estrogen and other hormones have a right to know how the medication is to be taken and what side effects can be anticipated. They should also be told how they can handle side effects of medication and what options are available. Cost of medication is an important factor especially when women pay for medication out of their pockets. Compliance to hormone therapy would improve if the patient is comfortable with many of the facts mentioned above.

Estrogen can either be orally or by non-oral routes.

ORAL ESTROGENS

Synthetic estrogen have been used commonly in low doses in contraceptive pills for well over 80 years. Contraceptive pills are not suitable as hormone therapy in the menopause. Naturally occurring estrogen like CONJUGATED EQUINE ESTROGEN (Premarin) became popular in the 1970s as hormone therapy. Since then a variety of other preparations are available. Once consumed orally the drug is slowly absorbed and circulates in the blood system after being processed in the liver.

Medication Regimes

Whenever estrogen therapy is prescribed one needs to consider the effect it has on the endometrium of the uterus. If prescribed continuously estrogen tends to also affect the endometrium of the uterus making it grow in thickness. This stimulatory effect is not desired. Hence women who have their uterus intact i.e have not had hysterectomy done, should also take progestogen to counteract the uninhibited growth of endometrium under the influence of estrogen. A minimum period of 12-14 days of progestogen should be added to the estrogen which may be taken for 21-28 days in a month.

Adding 12-14 days of progestogen literally opposes the continued effect estrogen has on the endometrium, hence preventing the potential development of pre-cancerous changes of the endometrium. The duration and preparation of progestogen varies according to the woman's needs.

In women who have an intact uterus are prescribed estrogen and progestogen, the hormone may be taken continuously as a 'no bleed regime' or for 21 days when a 'withdrawal bleed' is to be expected. The choice of regime will depend on how comfortable woman is. When the 'bleed regime 'is used, bleeding from the uterus is often scantier than normal menstruation. Some women are happy with the continuous regime as they do not want to have 'bleeding' after having attained menopause. Others may be happy with the bleed regime as they are free of having to take medication for 7 of the 28 days in a cycle.

The medication regime where estrogen is taken for 28 days per cycle without a drug free interval, progestogen need to be compulsorily added for about 12-14 days.

Should the patient have had a hysterectomy (surgical removal of the uterus) there is no risk of endometrium growing 'unabated' or 'unopposed'. Such women may take estrogen without having to add progestogen to the hormone regime (continuous regime).

Role of the Liver in Hormone Therapy

Any medication that is absorbed from the gut following oral administration enters the blood circulation undergoing metabolic changes in the cells of the liver and eventually excreted largely through the kidneys. The liver plays a very important role in metabolism of estrogen and other sex hormones. This central role liver plays has implications in both the good effects estrogen exerts and also 'bad effects'. When oral estrogen goes through the liver after absorption, it is called the FIRST PASS EFFECT. Such a phenomenon does not operate if estrogen was administered through other routes like application to the skin as patches.

The liver is the principal site for conjugation of estrogen (one of the vital cellular reactions). It is responsible for excretion (removal) and re-absorption of estrogen from bile, produces certain proteins called 'sex binding globulin' and determines how much of the dose of estrogen administered is truly available for use by body tissues. The liver is also involved in both carbohydrate and lipid metabolism and synthesis of coagulation (blood clotting) factors.

The effects on lipid metabolism may be summarised by stating that orally administered estrogen have a favourable effect on lipid metabolism. High density cholesterol (HDL-C) is seen to be favourably increased with a fall in low density cholesterol (LDL-C). These were reasons why estrogen was considered to have a good effect in preventing coronary heart disease after menopause. However more research is being done to address the true effects estrogen has in preventing coronary heart disease. The subject is discussed in Chapter 5. Epidemiological data shows the protective effect estrogen has in women on plaque formation in blood vessels.

A negative aspect of orally administered estrogen is its potential for increasing coagulability of blood making women vulnerable to deep vein thrombosis and strokes.

ESTROGENS TAKEN THROUGH NON-ORAL ROUTE

We have discussed about the most common means of taking estrogen i.e through the oral route and also mentioned about the role of the liver in metabolising the hormone after consumption. Some patients prefer non-oral route of administration of estrogen. Women need to be counselled on the benefits and risk of whatever route is opted for.

Whilst orally administered estrogen remains popular, applying the hormone to the skin and inserting it into the vagina are other options. The 'first pass effect' through the liver that was mentioned when estrogen is consumed orally is completely by—passed when the hormone is not taken by mouth.

There are instances where the oral route is contra-indicated, hence having alternative means of taking the hormone is sensible. One of such a reason could be the need for taking hormones in the presence of liver impairment.

Women requiring estrogen therapy should also be well informed of the various choices currently available in non-oral route of administration. She should be given the preferred choice for better compliance to medication.

Research on estrogen therapy aims to achieve the optimum dose titrated against relief of symptoms when hormone therapy is indicated. Current views are that there must be definite indications for use and lowest possible dose be prescribed. Such an approach should not only make the woman comfortable with improvement of quality of life but also appreciate that untoward effects will be minimized.

The two main routes of administering non-oral estrogen i.e application to the skin and inserting into the vagina will be discussed. A variety of proprietary applications are available. These include:

- Patch, Extended Release
- Gel/Jelly
- Spray
- Emulsion

i. Skin applications

a. *Oestradiol Implants*

Although injectable preparations of estrogen are available, IMPLANTS of ESTRADIOL became popular in the 1990s as they could be inserted and left under the skin surface. The active hormone is 17-beta- oestradiol which is incorporated into small pellets about 0.3 cm in diameter. These pellets are injected under the skin (subdermally) usually in the lower part of the abdomen or buttocks. A single pellet contains about 20-25 mg of 17-beta-oestradiol which releases the hormone slowly over a period of 8 weeks to 6 months depending on the preparation. About 0.1 mg of the hormone is released each day.

The advantage of this method of estrogen administration is that it is convenient as one does not have to remember taking the tablet each day. However, if the woman has an intact uterus she has to take about 12-14 days of progestogen in addition to estrogen for reasons mentioned. The disadvantage of subcutaneous implants is the difficulty in adjusting the required dose of medication especially if side effects are reported. It is also difficult to predict the end—point effectiveness of the hormone.

Practical hints on hormone implants

A mould holds fine crystals of the hormone. The hormone is slowly released into the blood circulation. Heat will increase absorption and hence should not be directly applied. Avoid hot water bottles from coming in contact with site of insertion. When there is fibrosis around skin there will less release of hormone.

b. Oestradiol Transdermal Patch

ESTRADERM is one of the transdermal patches available which uses what is called a 'CLOSED SYSTEM' in delivering estrogen into the blood circulation. A patch containing estrogen is available as 0.025 mg, 0.05 mg and 0.1 mg. The 0.05mg concentration delivers about 50 µg per 24 hours.

The hormone (estrogen) is contained in a reservoir with alcohol incorporated in a small adhesive patch. The hormone is released in a controlled manner through micropores in the ethylene acetate co-polymer membrane in the patch. The patch is usually placed on the buttocks and changed every 4 days (see the instructions on the preparation for details). An alternative to this is to use the patch for three weeks in a row with one week off.

Skin serves to absorb estrogen into the blood circulation without significantly going through the liver (first pass effect). Hence the estrogen administered this way has little effect on proteins (globulin). The beneficial effects of alleviating menopausal symptoms and preventing osteoporosis is sustained whatever the route of administration.

Skin patches of estrogen have not been tolerated by some women because of skin reactions. In the West about 20% of women are known to discontinue because of redness and itchiness following patch application. Women who prefer this mode of application are comfortable with it as it avoids having to take the hormone orally.

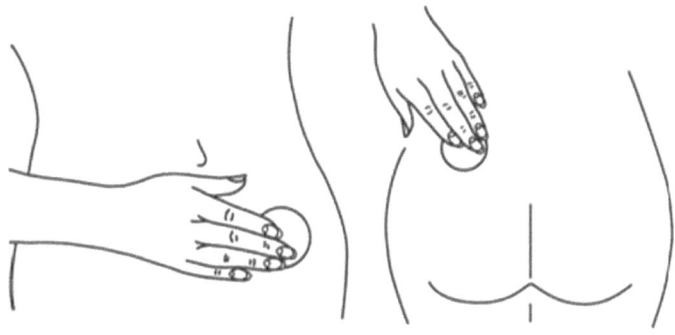

Fig. 11.2 Estrogen skin patch
(Avoid applying on the breast)

Percutaneous Oestradiol Gel

Percutaneous oestradiol gel (OESTROGEL, DIVIGEL) consist of oestradiol with alcohol. The preparation comes as a body lotion and is applied liberally over the arms and shoulder covering about 700 sq. cm of skin area on a daily basis. The lotion dries quickly after 2-5 minutes without any residue. The hormone is absorbed into the blood circulation though the skin and subcutaneous fat.

ii. Vaginal applications

The surface of the vagina absorbs estrogen very well. A variety of vaginal preparations are now available in the market. This mode of application does not appeal to some women.
Three preparations that are available include:

- Vaginal creams
- Vaginal Tablets
- Vaginal rings impregnated with estrogen
  - Vaginal creams
  - Vaginal Tablets
  - Vaginal estrogen bearing rings

Vaginal Cream

Both 17 β-oestradiol and conjugated equine estrogen creams are available as vaginal cream preparation. Vaginal cream preparation is popular in women who complain of painful sexual intercourse because of vaginal dryness and ATROPHIC VAGINITIS.
The cream is easy to apply with an applicator. Some find it 'messy; especially when it has to be applied frequently on a regular basis.

Vaginal Tablets

Tablets of 1 mg oestradiol (ESTRACE) can be placed high up the vagina and produce similar effects as vaginal cream.

Vaginal Rings Impregnated with Estrogen

'Polysiloxane' vaginal rings impregnated with oestradiol is placed high up the vagina like a contraceptive diaphragm. These rings may be left in the vagina for up to 3 months depending on the dose of estrogen. It does not interfere with sexual intercourse and is a good alternative to taking estrogen orally, daily. Rings bearing both estrogen and progestogen is now available particularly useful for those who still have the uterus intact.

Some precautions when taking medical hormone therapy

- If nausea is troublesome take medication with or after food. In most instances nausea disappears after the first few weeks
- Wash hand dry if skin patches are being used and apply patch to clean dry area of skin, preferably over lower part of abdomen, below waist or buttocks where there is little or no hair. Overlying clothes must be loose.
- New patch should be applied on a new site so that there is week free interval to reduce skin irritation.
- Follow instructions given when using emulsions
- Do not apply on breast

Alternatives to Medical Estrogen Therapy

Some women should not be prescribed estrogens e.g history of breast cancer. When these women are severely disturbed by vasomotor symptoms (hot flashes etc), alternative medication have been suggested if conventional advice fails. Medication used for treating depressive illness called SSRIs have been popular in such situations. These medication need a prescription by a doctor. Apart from relief of hot flashes, which should be experienced within a week of taking the medication, SSRIs also help in treating depression. As advised for all medication, only the lowest effective does is given. Side effects include nausea and even loss of sexual dysfunction. The two popular SSRIs are paroxetine and fluoxetine. Research shows moderate reduction in hot flashes of about 20% compared to placebos.

Another group of medication that have been researched on is venlafaxine. This is a drug that has a combination of serotonin and norepinephrine reuptake inhibitor. Reduction of hot flashes are seen with its use four weeks in randomised controlled trials. Again side effects with this medication that have been reported are nausea, dizzy spells, loss of sexual drive and constipation.

Gabapentin is another option which showed some effectiveness (51% VS, 26% reduction in hot flashes compared to placebo) when 900mg was prescribed for four weeks continuously. Side effects like dizziness and drowsiness improved after two weeks of use.

The use of alternative medication will require care consideration by doctors and current guidelines on their use must be sought.

Conclusion

Oral preparations of estrogen remain the most popular among women requiring hormone therapy. Alternative delivery routes like those that can be applied to the skin of the vagina may appeal to women who cannot tolerate the oral route or where if there is liver derangement. Women need to be counselled on the risk and benefits of hormone therapy and the cost effectiveness of each type of preparation that best suits them. Individual variations and patient preference are important in selecting a particular preparation of hormone therapy. It has been conclusively shown that hormone therapy alleviates menopausal symptoms especially hot flashes, night sweats and vaginal dryness which makes sexual intercourse painful.

Risk of endometrium growing abnormally is a voided by adding progestogen to the estrogen regime. The increased rate of breast cancer with long term use of estrogen therapy has been a troubling finding from epidemiological studies. This subject is discussed in detail in Chapter 17.

There is a definite role for taking short term hormone therapy without fear of adverse events in treating vasomotor symptoms and vaginal dryness. Alternatives to estrogen therapy are prescribed for vasomotor symptoms after careful consideration by the attending doctor.

CHAPTER 12

HORMONE MEDICAL THERAPY

Overcoming some related problems

As our generation of women become better educated as a result of better media coverage and access through the internet together with personal experiences gained from taking hormonal contraceptive pills in earlier life, a situation would arise when the demand for hormone therapy would be increase. The current guidelines on hormone therapy clearly indicate that prolonged use of hormones is not advisable. Physicians may vary in their approach to willingness to prescribe hormone therapy after the release of results of major clinical trials indicating a small increase in number of invasive breast cancer after prolonged use of hormone therapy. There is differing practice habits among medical practitioners regarding hormone therapy. A survey in Norway showed that younger physicians and female doctors were more prone to discuss hormone therapy compared to male physicians and their older colleagues. With an increasing number of women successfully achieving the climacteric due to increased longevity of life and with an massive increase in information access on the subject to both physicians and women, more women would seek hormone therapy to relieve troubling symptoms and to achieve maximum health benefit in preventing osteoporosis. Adherence to expert views and current guidelines would be preferred so as not to give conflicting views and suggestion leaving the client to make a decision about treatment options.

Current medical opinion is that medical hormone therapy is best to be prescribed in the lowest dose that would be necessary to relief menopausal symptoms for the shortest period. Menopausal symptoms that one is referring to are hot flashes, night sweats and dry vagina.

Compliance to hormone therapy

Chapter 22 deals with compliance with medical hormone therapy. Once there is an indication for hormone therapy, compliance to medication is vital for maximum benefit. All too often, when both the client and the attending physician are not sure of side-effects or troublesome effects of both disease and medication, the latter may be inadvertently stopped. When hormone therapy is a necessity, one should try to continue with therapy for a period of time as the body needs some time to adjust to the medication. A variety of problems are known to occur when on hormone therapy. Better compliance to medication is obtained if one is an aware of the possible adverse effects.

Three problems that are encountered which need elaboration are:

i. Persistence of symptoms
ii. Abnormal vaginal bleeding
iii. Side-effects

Persistence of Symptoms

Many patients have the wrong notion that once hormone therapy is prescribed, symptoms would immediately cease. Such a view is wrong and should not be reason for stopping medication before achieving the beneficial effects.

When clients do not benefit from medication one question that should be raised is, 'Is she getting the correct dose of hormone?'

Hormones prescribed for the menopause are available in specified formulation and need to be prescribed according to the constitution of the individual. Not all women respond in a uniform way to the prescribed dose. Allowance must be made for this fact. When hot flashes and night sweats are considered, the usual drug formulation prescribed could be 0.3 mg conjugated equine estrogen or 25 micrograms of transdermal oestradiol. Such a dose is adequate in most instances when women get about 6 episodes of hour flashes a day or about 2-3 episodes of night sweats. However, when symptoms persist for over three weeks, then a higher does may be required before withdrawing the hormone thinking that it is not effective. It is commonly mentioned that maximum relief of symptoms is not to be expected till duration of about three months has gone by.

When the dosage of the hormone appears okay, one is not sure how much is actually absorbed by the body. In a small number of women, taking the hormone by mouth (oral route) may not have achieved therapeutic levels in the body. The bowels may not absorb the entire drug consumed because of cross reaction with other medications or due to other factors that prevent normal absorption. In this respect, one should consider an alternative route with a different formulation like application on the skin or inserting an estrogen ring in the vagina.

One needs to bear in mind that hormones, like other prescriptive medications, can interact with other substances in the gut severely affecting their efficacy. One such medication is ANTIBIOTICS. Other prescription drugs implicated are barbiturates, anti-thyroid drugs, and anti-epileptic drugs. All those mentioned interfere with the metabolism of estrogen and prevent it reaching therapeutic levels.

Unfortunately, because of the protean nature of its presentation, climacteric or menopausal symptoms may not be truly associated with estrogen deficiency alone. For instances hot flashes are largely due to estrogen deficiency, and so is night sweats but when the menopausal woman complains of lethargy, joint pains and depression, these cannot be directly linked to estrogen deficiency. Other disorders like arthritis that comes with aging and obesity should be considered before hormones are considered. It is worthy of mention that failure to adequately counsel the woman prior to prescribing hormone therapy can lead to unrealistic expectations causing untold inconvenience and poor adherence to hormone therapy.

Abnormal Vaginal Bleeding

The menopausal woman who has not menstruated for some time must be warned of return of vaginal bleeds (withdrawal bleeding) if she had elected to go on the cyclical regime where there is a 7-day hormone free interval.

If the woman is taking hormones orally, she can expect to 'bleed vaginally' on the 10-11th day of adding the progestogen hormones or even later. Should she elect to be on skin patches, such withdrawal bleeding may occur earlier on the 8-9th day of initiating progestogen tablets.

Two types of abnormal vaginal bleeding are worth mentioning:

* Breakthrough bleeding
* Heavy and painful regular menstrual bleeding

Breakthrough bleeding occurs when hormones are not taken as advised resulting in inadequate dosage. Hormones are best taken regularly at prescribed times of the day. In the presence of vomiting due to any cause or if there is simultaneous need to take antibiotics, bioavailability of hormones is affected resulting in breakthrough bleeding. Stress factors and long distance travelling have also been implicated, though these need to be scientifically proven. Poor compliance to therapy is by far the main reason for alarming breakthrough bleeding especially when one is on the continuous combined regime.

Heavy bleeding and painful vaginal bleeding are symptoms that require a gynaecologist to review the woman and perform a thorough pelvic examination. Woman should be forewarned that withdrawal bleeding may be heavier if she is on the cyclical regime for the first one or two cycles but when symptoms persist for a longer period, one needs to exclude a gynaecological pathology. More often than not there is need to perform a hysteroscopic examination to look directly at the uterine cavity for polyps, fibroid or even a cancer.

If there is no pathology, reducing the dose of estrogen may be required. In some women they may be advised to have the uterine cavity treated with ENDOMETRIAL ABLATION by microwave energy or treating it with electrical cautery. Rarely, a hysterectomy may be advised to solve the problem of abnormal bleeding from the uterus before continuing estrogen therapy for relief of symptoms.

In some women who are on combined estrogen-progestogen hormone therapy, the problem may be due to insufficient dose of progestogen. So increasing the dose of progestogen and maintaining the same dose of estrogen would do the trick.

Side-effects

Side-effects due to hormone therapy have been a common reason for stopping the medication. Leg cramps have been reported though the cause is not known. Deep vein thrombosis is a complication that can occur with estrogen therapy but the clinical presentation is different. Breast tenderness is largely due to progestogens. A variety of both physical and psychological symptoms have been reported. Most of these appear to be worse when higher doses of progestogen are taken especially in those with pre-existing PREMENSTRUAL SYNDROME.

Administering the minimal dose of progestogen is recommended in those with the combined regime (to protect the endometrium). Changing the progestogen preparation to another may be tried. If the symptoms due to progestogen are severe, omitting the progestogen for three months before resuming the medication may be an option.

Some side-effects like dyspepsia may be due to oral hormones. One needs to exclude other causes of dyspepsia if the symptoms are severe or persistent. Nausea and dyspepsia due to oral medication may be less if the hormone is taken with food or at bedtime. If all these measures fail, one could try an alternative route other than the oral route.

Skin irritation with skin patches of estrogen has been reported. The alcohol that is incorporated should be allowed to evaporate from the patch before application. Rotating the site of application is also advised. Women with such a problem are advised against applying talcum powder or perfume to the area.

Weight gain is not due to estrogen hormone therapy and this fact needs emphasis. Neither does one develop high blood pressure because of estrogen hormone therapy.

CONCLUSION

The problems associated with hormone therapy are many but in most instances they are minor and not all women taking hormones have these complaints. Current information on side-effects and early consultation with your doctor is advisable as medication regimes need to be individualized. Compliance to medication improves with correct and sufficient knowledge on how hormones work and how some of the side-effects may be overcome. Convenient dosing and ease of administration of hormone are important for improved compliance to medication. Persistent and annoying symptoms like abnormal vaginal bleeding warrant further investigations by a gynaecologist. Above all there should be open channels for women to consult and discuss at all times about problems associated with hormone therapy ,apart from normal consultation hours, so as clarify issues related to hormone therapy and to encourage adherence to prescription regimes.

CHAPTER 13

ADHERENCE TO ESTROGEN THERAPY

'Adherence' to medication is now replacing the previous term 'compliance' frequently used in medical jargon. Adhering to estrogen (or hormone) therapy refers to whether the woman is taking her medication as prescribed as well as whether she continues to take for the duration prescribed. It would be difficult for clinicians and healthcare providers to determine if the person taking the medication is benefitting from hormone therapy and if there are adverse effects that need to be reported as a result of medication prescribed unless they are informed about such information by women taking the hormones.

Some of the common problems known are not following correct regime, not taking it at regular intervals, missing either taking tablets or not applying skin applications as advised and not adhering to the duration of medication that has been advised. Poor adherence to medication is difficult to evaluate. However, clinicians need to detect lack of adherence to medication, be able to detect such behaviour, find reasons for non-adherence and be conversant in advising women on issues related to non-adherence.

Previous research studies have shown that about 40 % of women prescribed estrogen therapy do not adhere to prescription orders.

Why is estrogen therapy indicated

Endocrine deficiency results in disease. Diabetes mellitus occurs when the pancreas does not produce adequate amount of insulin preventing blood sugar from entering the tissues and cells. Treatment would be stimulating the pancreas to produce more insulin with medication or to replace the body with adequate amounts of insulin by injections. Similarly if the thyroid gland does not produce sufficient thyroxine producing symptoms related to that hormone, clinicians would prescribe oral tablets of THYROXINE. Patients respond to replacement therapy rapidly and continue to enjoy improved quality of life with life long replacement therapy.

Can a similar approach be taken with women who reach menopause and suffer the problems related to menopause? That was the rationale when estrogen replacement therapy was initially popularised. Women prescribed estrogen found a marked rejuvenation effect with positive changes in their skin, vagina as well as relief of menopausal symptoms. Surgically induced menopause as a result of both ovaries being removed for gynaecological reasons resulted in menopausal symptoms occurring much earlier especially if the surgery had been performed between 40-50 years. Estrogen therapy became the saviour in these women who suffer disabling menopausal symptoms.

Based on scientific research and clinical studies, estrogen therapy can prevent osteoporosis, relieve climacteric symptoms (hot flashes, night sweat etc), improve psychosexual disturbances and are effective in treating urogenital atrophy. However, despite these favourable effects of estrogen therapy concerns have been expressed about increased risks of invasive breast cancer, myocardial infarction and coronary thrombosis, deep vein thrombosis and strokes when used in specific groups of women. Contradictory reports of increases in the blood clotting system and untoward effects on endometrium and breast have been cited as reason for non-adherence to estrogen therapy. Women need clear and non-confusing information on the safety profile of estrogen therapy. Side-effects like breast pain and undesired uterine bleeding while on estrogen can be perplexing and uncomfortable. How should such problems be predicted and managed are vital discussion points which would affect adherence to medication.

The problems related to estrogen therapy are not quite the same as life-long insulin therapy for diabetes mellitus and thyroxine therapy for hypothyroidism. Other factors like old age, co-morbid disease like pre-existing coronary thrombosis, obesity, hypertension and diabetes need to be considered when long term estrogen therapy is to be considered. The Women's Health Initiative (WHI) study has cautioned the long term use of estrogen and progestogen. In that longitudinal study of 160 000 women between 50-79 years taking estrogen with progestogen were recruited and followed up for several years. Women on estrogen and progestogen were more likely to develop invasive breast cancer apart from some the conditions mentioned above. The results of the study released in 2002 and 2004, impacted on prescription behaviour and the number of women electing to go on hormone therapy declined. The findings of the study have been debated in medical circles stating that the increased rate of invasive breast cancer, coronary heart disease, stroke and deep vein thrombosis were because women recruited were older, obese and had chronic diseases.

Two other studies appear to report more favourable results with less risk if the estrogen therapy was initiated early after onset of menopause. The KEEP's study involved 727 women while a Danish study involving 1006 women aged 45-58 years, had a longer follow up of 16 years compared to the KEEPS study. The latter study emphasizes the importance of 'transition hypothesis' as an important factor as women were around the menopause age when hormones were prescribed. At the end of 10 years of follow up, there was a 52% reduction in myocardial infarction or heart failure with no associated increase in any cancer.

Do side-effects contribute to drug non-adherence?

The Nurse's Health Study in the US is considered the 'grandmother' of all health studies done on women. Started in 1976 and expanded in 1989, it led to understanding of health and disease. It provided information on associated factors contributing to cancer, cardiovascular disease, diabetes and several other conditions. Although it was an observational study it revealed some pertinent facts like modification of diet, increasing physical activity and avoiding smoking contributed to lower rates of disease. When hormone therapy was evaluated, only 17% postmenopausal continued to take medication for at least 8 years.

One of the unpleasant effects of hormone therapy is withdrawal bleeding from the uterus. The cessation of menstruation is accepted by most women at menopause. Certain cultures and religious groups (Muslim, Hindu) appreciate this transition from reproductive age to menopausal life as it would permit them to visit places of worship without interruption and hindrance.

Summarily stated there are various reasons why women do not adhere to prescribed drugs. Some of those relevant to hormone therapy are listed below and will be discussed in turn.

- Withdrawal Uterine Bleeding

- Vaginal Spotting
- Breast Discomfort and Breast Tenderness
- Fear of Cancer
- Ill-informed or Lack of Information

a. Withdrawal Uterine Bleeding

Withdrawal uterine bleeding is only an issue in women who have an intact uterus i.e those who have not had a hysterectomy done. Women prescribed cyclical hormones with a 7 day drug free interval would be taking 21 days of estrogen with about 12-14 days of progestogen. Such patients may welcome the 7 day drug-free interval in each month of hormone therapy improving adherence to medication treatment or drug adherence. Withdrawal bleeding from the uterine cavity can be anticipated in such women. They should be counselled on this 'resumption' of menstruation' because of hormone therapy. They need to be further evaluated for pathology in the genital tract should the 'menstrual bleeding' not be regular or predictable during the seven day drug free interval before continuation of such a regime.

Should they express displeasure at withdrawal uterine bleeding, they should be offered alternatives like 'continuous hormone regime' where no drug free interval is present. Progestogens are added to estrogen therapy for 12-14 days to protect the endometrium of the uterus from unopposed effects of estrogen. Alternative way of prescribing progestogen would be by inserting a progestogen bearing intrauterine contraceptive device (LEVONOGESTREL—MIRENA).

In most women, withdrawal bleeding is predictable and regular. They are advised to seek medial consultation should the bleeding not be regular.

b. In Vaginal Spotting

Another objectionable symptom is little 'bits' of bleeding called SPOTTING which occurs at various intervals while the woman is on hormone therapy. Many a time it is unpredictable. While the body needs to adjust to the correct dose in the beginning, such symptoms should rarely persist for longer than three months of beginning hormone therapy. Should such symptoms persist she needs to be evaluated. One should enquire into drug adherence and timing of drug administration daily. When a woman take hormones regularly as prescribed, effective levels of hormones are reached in the blood so as to not adversely affect the endometrium leading to undesired bleeding. Should hormone levels fall below a certain threshold, there is a risk of 'spotting'. Close questioning of the symptoms and a change in formulation of the hormones would overcome troublesome spotting.

Say for example, a woman is taking a dose of 0.625 mg Premarin daily, regularly and follows the regime prescribed for progestogen tablets and yet has spotting, there could be several reasons for this. As mentioned, spotting may occur in the first few months as the body 'titrates' to the appropriate levels of the hormones. However, if the absorption of the hormone is a problem then the amount of hormone circulating in the blood is affected leading to an issue of BIOAVAILABILITY and effectiveness. In such situations a higher dose of the hormone may be required. Another option may be for the need to increase the dose of progestogen. If such measures do not work, an alternative hormone regime may have to be prescribed. Such alternatives may be estrogen implant, estrogen vaginal ring or skin preparations of estrogen.

Having said that, as mentioned earlier, should this abnormal bleeding persist, the clinician would also look for pathology in the genital tract or some other cause that is not permitting the hormone to be effectively functioning. Most women who are started on hormone therapy would have had a complete physical examination including genital tract evaluation so as to exclude pre-existing gynaecological pathology. This is periodically done after initiating hormone therapy for as long as she is on treatment as part of 'well women' examination.

c. Breast Discomfort and Breast Tenderness

MASTODYNIA refers to breast pain, breast tenderness and breast discomfort. As estrogen has a direct effect on breasts, these symptoms are not uncommon. Sometimes when the symptoms are extreme one should suspect if bioavailable estrogen levels in blood circulation and relevant tissues are high. When women have these symptoms, suitable changes should be made to drug dosage. Current views are that the lowest effective dose of estrogen should only be prescribed.

For effective hormone levels, estrogen levels need to be about 60 pg/ml. Despite getting optimum relief of hot flashes, achieving protective effect on bone and preventing dry vagina, if levels are extremely high (>160pg/ml) she may experience mastodynia.

d. Fear of Cancer

Fear of cancer has been a common reason for not adhering to prescribed regimes or not wanting to continue estrogen for prolonged periods exceeding years. Women are known to manipulate the dosing of estrogen by taking less or not taking them daily, hoping to decrease the risk of cancer of the breast and endometrium. Some are happy with short term therapy if the primary complaint was hot flashes and this did not persist as a problem after a few months of hormone therapy.

Much should be left to the needs and wishes of the women but she should be cautioned of withdrawal uterine bleeding (in those with intact uterus) and this could be due insufficient dosing of hormones.

It would be comforting to women if they understood the need to titrate the drug dose according to each individual's body habitus and that the lowest effective dose would be maintained. It is no longer an acceptable belief that one should try to mimic the natural levels of hormones in the body of women in the reproductive age group. It has been agreed that levels between 60-80 pg/ml is sufficient to derive beneficial effects.

e. Ill-informed women and lack of information

It is common teaching that women rarely would adhere to hormone therapy if they are ill-informed or are confused as much literature is available in media giving both beneficial and adverse effects of hormone therapy. The internet has been a source of information and the availability of numerous proprietary drugs together with numerous alternatives to hormone (BIOIDENTICAL HORMONES, Fig. 21.1) can be confusing. Many women do not have a clear understanding of the hormones involved in menstruation and what happens to the genital tract at the time of menopause. Providing women information that is correct and current with suitable alternatives is essential.

Consultations need to answer queries and should not be rushed. Menopause is a transition in life and several issues apart from hormone therapy need to be discussed. Public talks, input by social workers and information in plain language would improve dissemination of correct information pertaining to hormone therapy.

Individualizing hormone therapy to improve drug-adherence

Some reasons for not adhering to hormone therapy has been discussed above. An old observational study in Paris in 1990 evaluated 179 women who were on oestradiol gel (skin application) and were analysed after a year of prescription. The average age of women was 62 years. Only 15.6 % were following the regime as advised. The main reasons for non-adherence to medication were:

- Conflicting recommendations by physicians

- Fear of breast cancer
- Fear of weight gain
- Skin irritation

Although this is an old study which does not meet the rigour of a randomized research trial, two vital points are illustrated:

- Physician's differing views on hormone therapy
- Acceptability of mode of administration of estrogen and proprietary type

While we continue to discuss the availability of correct information using lay language to women and their complete understanding of the transition to menopause, clinicians themselves need to have current knowledge and consensus views on hormone therapy. The subject has been debated for the last three decades and prescribing habits may differ between health providers. Giving conflicting advice can be confusing and disturbing especially when short course of estrogen for menopausal symptoms has been accepted as standard of care in those with severe menopausal symptoms.

The varying acceptability of certain hormone formulations is a known reason for non drug-adherence. Some women deliberately cease oral tablets of hormone because of minor symptoms like breast tenderness and nausea. Alternative routes to oral administration like skin preparations of estrogen may be a better option in such instances.

The duration of estrogen administration has implications. Menopausal symptoms, if present would require estrogen therapy for periods of 6 months to 2 years. Should one target osteoporosis prevention, long term use of estrogen would be required. There is a need to closely follow current guidelines in prescribing medical hormone therapy with regards to indications, duration and dose so as to assist women to both adhere to prescription and also benefit from medical hormone therapy.

Conclusion

Adherence to estrogen and progesterone therapy is a very individual matter. A discussion on menopause and its effects should go beyond hormone prescription with enquires into acceptability of side effects, preferred route of administration and cost-benefit. Hormone therapy is beneficial for menopausal symptoms and quality of life improves. Non-adherence to hormone therapy could be due to several reasons which include misinformation, fear of cancer and troubling side-effects. Clinicians would need to assist women by enquiring into reasons for non-adherence and offer change of dose of medication or alternate routes of administration.

Non-hormonal approaches in managing menopausal symptoms like balanced diet, exercise, relief of stress factors and physical exercise are equally important. The take home message for hormone therapy is adequate counselling, individualizing prescription of hormone regimes, adjusting dosage of hormones in presence of side-effects and clearly stating the duration of hormone therapy required for the woman. One needs to always find the reason women do not adhere to drug prescription!

Source:

1. Kroon's Longevity Research Institute. Hormone therapy has many favourable effects in newly menopausal women: Initial findings of the Kronos Early Estrogen Prevention Study (KEEPS) [press release]. October 3, 2012
2. Schierbeck LL et al. Effect of hormone replacement therapy on cardiovascular events in recently postmenopausal women: randomised trial BMJ2012;345doi:http://dx.doi.org/10.1136/bmj. e6409(Published 9 October 2012)
3. *Source: Highlights of Nurse's Health Study Summarized:*
    http://www.channing.harvard.edu/nhs/?page_id=197

CHAPTER 14

ROLE OF PROGESTERONE—
the other female hormone

Throughout the discussion on menopause reference has been made to estrogen deficiency as the primary defect after menopause. The menstrual cycle involves a chain of events initiated from the brain, ovaries and uterine cavity (endometrium). Synchronous discharge of all hormones concerned in menstrual cycle is essential for release of an ovum from the ovary and preparation of the uterine cavity (endometrium). Estrogen alone is not sufficient for this efficient system. Other hormones are involved and one of the more important hormones is progesterone.

Progestogens are synthetic hormones functioning like natural progesterone hormone and have equal or higher potency. Progesterone is chemically derived from C-19 steroids and C-21 steroids. The former (C-19 steroids) apparently exert some minimal effects likened to the male hormone, testosterone. Pure progesterone does not have this effect but are too expensive to be commercially produced. Synthetic progesterone's (progestogen) are in common use for hormone therapy.

A simple discussion on the role of female hormones and their effects on menstruation (Fig.14.1) appear in Chapter 1. Much more needs to be considered in understanding the role and effect of each of the hormones and chemical substances on target organs in the reproductive system. However, this is beyond the scope of this book. A detailed description of the menstrual cycle including the integral role progesterone plays is reviewed here for readers.

Menstruation and the influence of Hormones

Two organs at the base of the brain, the hypothalamus and the pituitary glands, regulate the functioning ovaries through a feedback mechanism. The ovaries respond to pituitary hormones by producing estrogen and progesterone. The latter act on the endometrium to help it grow in thickness (see Fig.14.1). After menopause when the ovaries atrophy, the estrogen levels fall markedly and do not stimulate the endometrium causing it to atrophy accounting for the cessation of regular menstrual bleeding. The feedback mechanism to the brain also fails leading to very high levels of gonadotrophin (elevated FSH, diagnostic of menopause).

The hypothalamus is involved in production of a preparatory hormone called Gonadotrophin Releasing Hormone (GnRH) which is released into the blood circulation within the pituitary gland, called the master gland. A variety of other hormones are produced by the pituitary apart from FSH and LH hormones (gonadotrophin).

The ovary has different types of cells in addition to follicles which eventually mature to become the ovum (egg). One type of cell is called THECA INTERNA which is regulated by LH. Another type of cell of importance in the ovary is GRANULOSA cells. The latter are stimulated by FSH. The female's hormones estrogen and progesterone are produced through a complicated pathway involving specific enzymes.

As mentioned estrogen has multiple functions including the feedback mechanism in regulating the release of gonadotrophin. In a rather complicated way estrogen and gonadotrophin also play pivotal roles in inducing the production of progesterone. Fig.14.1 shows the fluctuating levels and relationship between gonadotrophin and estrogen/progestogen.

Progesterone and Menopause

Let's recollect what happens when women approach the menopause. Ovaries have a definite life span and will lose most of their function with menopause. The female fetus has about seven million immature oocytes (potential eggs). Many of these fail to survive. At birth the female child probably has only about a million of these immature oocytes. When they attain puberty only about 400 000 remain for reproductive function. During each menstrual cycle, many potential oocytes are recruited (perhaps about 20 each month). Only one is mature enough for fertilization.

What happens at menopause? The ovaries are exhausted of most viable oocytes and begin to atrophy. Anovulation follows (i.e no ova are released). At this stage the levels of estrogen decline rapidly to 40-60% but progesterone levels fall to indeterminable levels. There appears to be a disproportion in the decline of these two hormones. During the reproductive years, progesterone played a regulatory role in balancing the action of estrogen and also improving the efficiency of action of estrogen on various tissues especially the endometrium and breast. This fine balance between the two primary hormones is no longer held after menopause.

Action of Estrogen and Progesterone on the Uterus

The endometrium, the inner lining of the uterus close to the cavity of the uterus, responds to both estrogen and progesterone and facilitates its preparation for pregnancy. If fertilization does not occur, menstruation results as the hormones do not sustain the thickened endometrium.

Oestradiol, the active form of estrogen, has several effects on the endometrium. It stimulates the endometrial cells to grow, permitting rapid multiplication (myogenic). At the same time it also prepares the endometrial cells to respond appropriately to the action of progesterone.

Progesterone acts opposite to estrogen and this action is beneficial to the endometrium in not permitting the action of estrogen to go unabated resulting in abnormal proliferation of the endometrium. The latter action can result in abnormal thickening with no shedding of the endometrium. Some pathological changes seen in the endometrium where the estrogen action is rather longer than normal are endometrial hyperplasia, endometrial polyps and endometrial cancer. This is the reason why progestogen has to be added to the hormone therapy regime in women who have not had hysterectomy for a minimum of 12-14 days.

It could then be summarily stated that unopposed estrogen will cause endometrial cells to multiply unabated resulting in endometrial pathology. Progesterone's have an 'anti-estrogenic effect' on the endometrium. It goes on to say that women who have had a hysterectomy do not need progesterone to be added to estrogen therapy by virtue of not having a uterus.

PROGESTERONES AND ESTROGENS:
Chemical Structure

The chemical structure of estrogen and progesterone's is illustrated with androgens in Fig. 11.1

Without getting into the details of chemistry, the structure of the three main hormones (estrogen, progesterone and androgens), all are derived from a common base. There are but few stereo chemical differences in the carbon chains. This ought to be an important observation. Mention was made as to how specific enzymes can act on the hormones in transformation into other products with slightly different action on tissues.

Synthetically produced progesterone like NORETHISTERONE is derived from C-19 steroids which have a little of androgenic effect—a little like the effect of the male hormone, testosterone. Another formulation of progesterone (e.g. DYDRGESTERONE) is related to the C-21 steroid and slightly less androgenic effect.

ROLE OF PROGESTERONE

Drugs and medication that have progestogenic effect are referred to as PROGESTOGENS. Progestogens that have been synthetically produced are used in hormone therapy as they are stable for oral use. There are also other forms of progestogens like vaginal tablets, injectables and those that are incorporated into INTRAUTERINE DEVICES.

Common regimes for hormone therapy and when progestogen should be added to estrogen therapy has been discussed Chapter 11. In the 'bleed' regime the patient takes 21 days of estrogen with about 12-14 days of progestogen added on in the latter part of the regime. This would result in regular monthly bleeding and also protect the endometrium from over-stimulation by estrogen. In the 'no-bleed regime' there is no drug free interval but the duration of progestogen added remains the same (12-14 days).

Side-effects of Progestogens

All medications invariably have side effects. Most are tolerable while others need some drug manipulation and advice. Progestogen therapy is not different. When progestogen dose is too high for the woman, side-effects may be more apparent. Table 14.1 shows the common side-effects of progestogen.

Table 14.1: Side-effects of Progestogens

▪ Breakthrough per vaginal bleeding
▪ Nausea
▪ Breast tenderness
▪ Fluid retention
▪ Mood swings
▪ Depression

Side-effects are usually seen when hormones are first initiated. They tend to become tolerable over time. When women complain of abnormal bleeding which is not acceptable there may be a need to discuss compliance to medication and review the dose of estrogen and progestogen in the hormone regime prescribed. If the bleeding is a new complaint after a period of having been on the hormones, further investigations need to be done as indicated by preliminary physical examination and transvaginal ultrasound of the pelvis.

In cases of nausea women may need to be advised to take the medication at different times of the day. Breast tenderness, if present, tends to subside after a few cycles. If they persist one may need to consider alternatives like reducing the dose of progestogen. Individual variations are common and one needs to tailor the drug regime to best suit the client. Women who are aware of common but tolerable side-effects tend to adhere to continued medication so as to obtain best benefits and improvement of quality of life.

Conclusion

Synthetic progestogen in the lowest dose that is effective should be prescribed for hormone therapy. There are many formulations and most are combined with estrogen for ease of prescription. Progestogens are derived from C-19 steroids and C-21 steroids. When side effects become troublesome switching the formulations based on the type of steroid used may be of help.

Progestogen should be included in all regimes where estrogen hormone therapy is prescribed if the woman has not has a hysterectomy (intact uterus) to protect abnormal proliferation of the endometrium under the influence of estrogen.

Further Reading

http://www.livestrong.com/article/315275-what-are-the-functions-of-progesterone-in-menopause/#ixzz2KjTXIHqPurther reading

CHAPTER 15

THE ROLE OF THE MALE HORMONE IN MENOPAUSE

Historically, menopause was thought to be completely reversible with supplementation with female hormones especially estrogen. We now know that estrogen is effective in relief of symptoms related to the menopause. With greater understanding of the ageing process, it is clearer that other hormones like progesterone and the male hormones, collectively called ANDROGENS, also have roles to play in treating symptoms of menopause. We have seen the chemical structure of the three hormones which share a common basic structure and how specific enzymes are capable of changing the orientation of the chemical structure to produce differing substrates.

Interestingly, the androgens which are vital in expression of 'manliness' in the male, also has a small role to play in females. It is known fact that ovaries not only produce estrogen and progestogen but also androgens. Up to 50% of androgens in the female body are lost as ovaries cease functioning at menopause. This fact underscores the role androgens have in women.

Androgens in the Climacteric

Androgens can be formed and/or produced in three anatomical sites of the body:

i.   Adrenal glands
ii. Ovaries

iii. Fat (adipose) tissue

The amount or androgens produced by the ovaries is regulated by the hormone LH (Luteinizing hormone) and to some extent, FSH (Follicle stimulating hormone). Although the ovaries produce less androgen than adrenal glands, androgens from the ovaries are more potent. During the climacteric, androgen production declines markedly. However, there is continued release of androgens (testosterone, a potent androgen), though at a lower level.

Table 15.1 Types of Male Hormones in Women

Androgen (Male Hormone) (μgm/ml)	Reproductive Age	Post-menopausal	Ovaries removed (at surgery)
Androsteinedione	2-3	0.5-1.0	0.4-0.8
Dehydroiepiandrosteinedione	6-8	1.5-4.0	1.5-4.0
Dehydroiepiandrosteinedione sulphate	8-12	4.0-9.0	4.0-9.0
Testosterone	200-250	50-100	20-70

Testosterone is produced in the ground substance of the ovaries while the other androgens are from the follicles. With the onset of menopause, the follicles are depleted and so estrogen production declines more markedly than testosterone. In a woman who has both ovaries removed at surgery or has had radiation therapy to the pelvis all forms of androgens including testosterone decline (Table 15.1).

Let's recollect some facts about androgens:

- *Progesterone, androgens and estrogen are produced in the ovaries*
- *There are several types of androgens (four are noted in Table 15.1)*
- *The adrenal glands and other organs are central to production of androgens*
- *The three hormones in women are capable of structural changes through the action of specific enzymes*

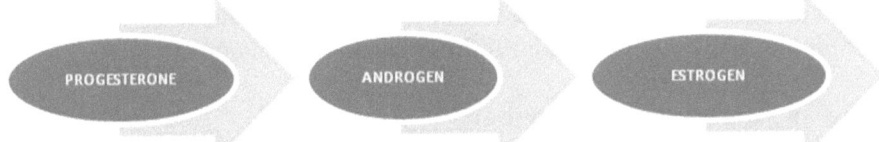

Fig. 15.1. Pathway of Hormone Conversion from one form to another

Although overall androgen production declines in menopause, the adrenal glands continue to produce small amounts of androgens with ageing. If the women have had a hysterectomy done well before natural menopause, decline in androgen production is much more rapid.

Role of Androgens in Women

We are now clear that all women produce androgens. Androgens may contribute to several physiological effects which won't be discussed in detail here. They include the maintenance of normal ovarian function, intellectual capacity, and sexual behaviour. As shown in Fig. 15.1 testosterone acts as a substrate for conversion to estrogen. Other androgens from the adrenal glands (Androsteinedione, DHEA and DHEAS) could be converted to testosterone and estrogen through enzymatic action.

Apart from the potential of enzymes to convert androgens to estrogen, their beneficial effects are explicitly demonstrated when androgens are administered together with conventional hormone therapy. A greater sense of well-being and higher energy levels are noted. Research also shows women felt less lethargic and tired.

Much controversy reigns as to specific signs of androgen deficiency in the menopause and should one prescribe androgens in addition to conventional hormone therapy. The FDA does not recommend addition of testosterone to hormone therapy. Common symptoms associated with androgen deficiency are loss of sexual function, diminished libido, depression, decreased bone and muscle mass.

The greatest advantage of adding androgen to estrogen therapy in earlier research was seen in psychological functioning. There were some positive changes in sexual functioning. Sexual arousal, improved and sexual desire and fantasy was increased to higher levels. An improvement in libido was also noted in research subjects.

One side-effect of adding androgens (especially when administered as and implant) is increased though mild growth of hair in the upper lips and chin (hirsutism). This annoying 'male effect' can be reduced or prevented by reducing the does or stopping androgen therapy for a while. Deepening if the voice is another side-effect when androgens should be stooped.

How is Androgens Prescribed?

Androgens are available as:

i.   Tablets
ii. Dermal patches
iii. Injectable
iv. Subcutaneous pellets

Oral tablet of 1.25mg or 2.5 mg methyl-testosterone is available in combination with estrogen. Injectable androgens come as DEPO-TESTOSTERONE in a dose of 50 mg/ml given once a month. Subcutaneous pellets come as 75 mg doses. These are implanted under the skin, each lasting for 4-6 months. Estrogen and progestogen therapy should follow suggested regimes.

Conclusion

Androgens appear to have a limited a role in managing women after the menopause. They are produced in the ovaries apart from other sites like the adrenals. Testosterone continues to be produced by ovaries, in smaller amounts after menopause. They influence sexual functioning and induce a state of well-being in women. Sexual desire and sexual arousal has been positively described due to the addition of androgens to conventional hormone therapy. As the role of testosterone in menopausal women is not conclusive, women should medical opinion.

Further reading

Somboonporn W. Androgen and menopause. Current Opinion in Obstetrics and Gynecology. 2006; 18(4); 427-423

CHAPTER 16

THE FEMALE BREAST
in health and disease

Despite wide publicity given to breast cancer, there remains continued reluctance to either perform 'self breast examination' or have their breasts examined by health care providers in developing countries. In certain communities general practitioners, especially male doctors, are reluctant to offer this service when the consultation was not related to breast ailment for fear of litigation. Occasional adverse publicity appearing in the media in respect to 'outrage of modesty' has contributed, to some extent, this change in practice. The rushed manner in which consultations are done focussing on primary problem presented no longer allocate time for discussion on 'wellness care' such as discussions on pap smear and breast examination. Current views today downplay the value of breast examination in detecting breast tumours. It is thought not to be an effective or sensitive test whether done by the woman or her physician. In the Americas there is a differing view between US and Canada on this matter.

The US Preventive Services Task Force found insufficient evidence from research to recommend for or against routine clinical examination to screen for breast cancer, or to recommend for or against teaching or performing routine breast self-examination. On the other hand the Canadian Task Force on Preventive Health Services recommends taking a more firm view against teaching self-examination to women aged 40 to 69 years due to "fair evidence of no benefit and good evidence of harm (Gaskie S, Nashelsky J. J.

Is self-exams or clinical exams effective for screening breast cancer? Family Practice 2005;54:9t)

Having said that we continue to advocate self-breast examination once a month as nearly 40% of lumps in the breasts is detected by women themselves. As breast cancer is the commonest tumor in women, any opportunistic encounter with a female should raise a discussion on breast health and screening modalities including self-breast examination. Health professionals in low resource countries or where screening with mammogram is not readily available would benefit from education on proper techniques of self-breast examination so as to sustain breast health awareness especially when one approaches menopause.

Breasts as part of the reproductive system

Medical knowledge clearly points to the breast being an integral part of the female reproductive system and is often implicated in health and disease. The female hormones influence the growth of the breasts in preparation for lactation and have a role to play in development of breast tumours. Certain varieties of tumors of the ovary and endometrium (uterine lining) are associated with breast cancer.

A discussion on the anatomy and physiological of the female breasts would be useful as several breast conditions, apart from breast cancer are known to occur throughout the reproductive age.

In medical terms the breast is referred to as the 'MAMMARY GLAND'. It develops under the influence of estrogen especially in adolescence till it reaches adult size. The mass of breast tissue is made of fat which helps breast to be firm. The breast is held firmly to the base by thickened fibres call fibrous tissue. Both breasts at attached to the muscles of the chest in front. The size and shape of the breast varies from individual to individual. Although both breasts develop uniformly from early development, it is not uncommon to notice some degree of asymmetry in women. It is pertinent to notice that the breast has a little tail end in it is upper outer quadrant which projects into the armpit (axilla). In performing breast examination the tail of the breast needs to be examined too.

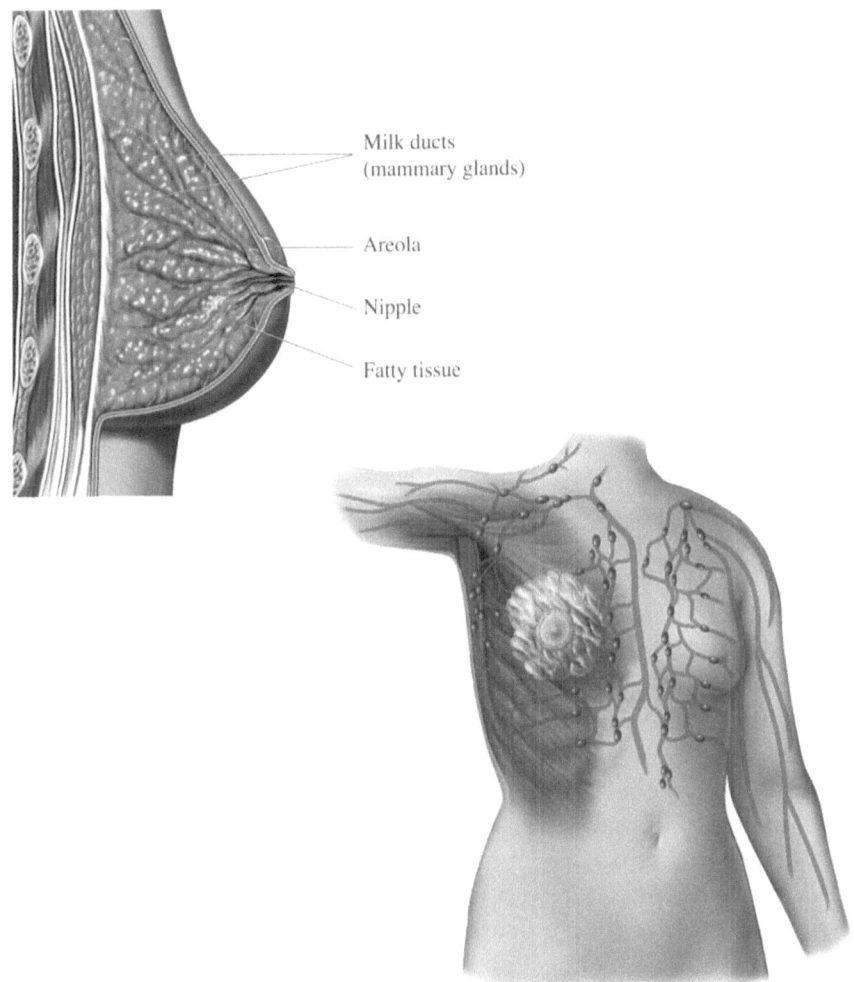

Fig.16.1 (a & b) The Female Breast (showing breast parts and lymphatic drainage)

In an adult woman, the breast contains about 15-20 lobes which consists of both fatty tissue and glandular tissue (referred to as TUBULO-ALVEOLAR GLANDS, Fig. 16.1). The glandular tissue, which lies under the skin of the breast, is a modified form of sweat gland which has the potential to expand and grow under the influence of female hormones. The breasts would shrivel and become smaller (involute) when estrogen becomes depleted at the time of menopause. The upper part of the breasts, especially the outer side, contains more glandular tissue than the rest of the breast. This is also the site for most of the breast cancers (Fig. 16.2)

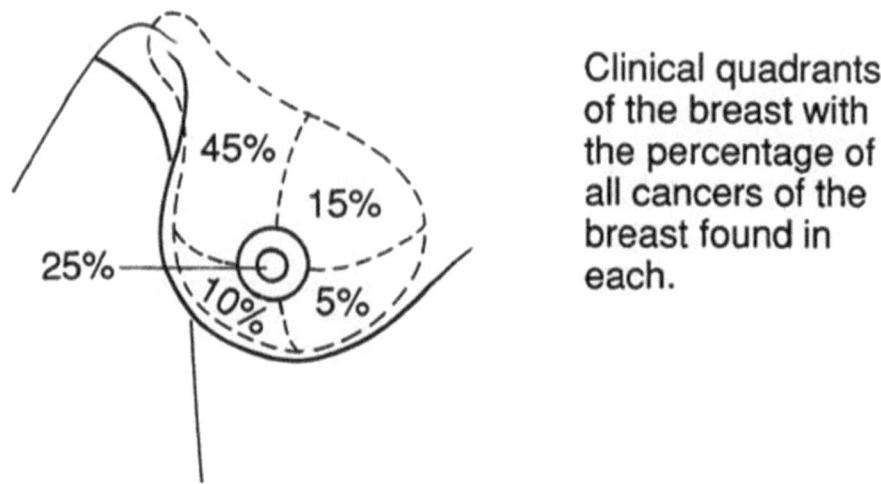

Fig.16.2 Prevalence of Cancer by Quadrant of Breast

Most of the bulkiness of the breast is due to fatty tissue. Age and hormonal status also influences state and development of breasts. The areola is a distinctly distinguishable circular darkened area on which the nipple is situated. It is usually about 3-5 cm in diameter. The nipple is darker and appears wrinkled and conical. It has the ability to become erect on stimulation.

The 15-20 'lobules' of the breast mentioned above, are arranged in a radial manner as if they are 'fanning' out to the rest of the breast. Each lobule is discrete and is separated from its neighbour by fibrous tissue. The space between lobules is filled in with fatty tissue (adipose tissue). As the lobule has gland bearing cells, fluid produced by these cells will exit though openings called DUCTS in the nipple. The glandular portion of breast bears a complex of milk producing structures called ALVEOLI. These are arranged like the branches and leaves or a tree. Milk, once produced, tracks along the ducts to be expelled at the nipple when a baby suckles it.

We have mentioned the size and shape of the breast are largely determined by the amount of fat and fibrous tissues. Hence more the number of fat cells, the larger the breast. The firmness of the breast is maintained by fibrous tissue permitting it to sag when they become lax.

The cells forming the ALVEOLI are under the influence of hormones and will produce milk when the woman becomes pregnant. Milk production and release from the breast are under the influence of prolactin and oxytocin, two vital hormones prominent in late pregnancy.

Glandular tissue grows larger as pregnancy advances preparing for lactation. During the first few days following childbirth breasts release

COLUSTRUM, a fluid very rich in antibodies, which protects the suckling baby from various infections. Milk production proper follows after release of colostrum. As the glandular tissue increase in size with milk production, some decrease in fat occurs with laxity of the fibres. The breasts become pendulous because of these changes.

Of particular importance to diseases of the breast are the blood supply and lymphatic system apart from the structures stated (Fig. 16.1). The lymphatic system runs close to the arteries and veins supplying the breast playing a vital defence mechanism against invasion by micro-organisms and cancer cells.

The blood vessels and lymphatics seen in the breast include:

- Perforating branches of the Internal Mammary vessels going through the muscles of the rib cage
- Axillary vessels which eventually communicate with great vessel reaching the heart
- Intercostal vessels which go through the chest wall in front

Importance of understanding the structure of the breast

Women become alarmed at symptoms related to the breast due to a lack of understanding of the anatomy and physiological changes that have been discussed. Although the primary role of the breasts is for milk production to feed the young, they are prone to disease in a few women. Disease may be confined to the skin overlying the breast including nipples. Abnormal discharge from the nipples, abnormalities of the glandular tissues especially in its response to female hormones and diseases of the fat and fibrous component may manifest in various ways. Women who regularly perform self breast examination would be familiar to the texture and feel of their breasts and be familiar with the clinical changes due to fluctuating levels of hormones in the body.

It is good advice to determine the consistency of the breasts by feeling the texture of both breasts after applying some soap during baths. The skin feels smooth. Any lumpiness or 'bumps' are best felt with the pads of the fingers. Nipples are usually everted or pout outwards. Some women may have 'inverted' nipples from childhood.

It would become easy for a woman who regularly examines her breasts to be able to detect changes in the breast. Any doubts should be cleared by a visit to the doctor. The term "benign breast diseases" includes a heterogeneous group of conditions presenting with a wide range of symptoms. The use of mammograms and MRI have increased detection rates of benign disease without symptoms. Benign breast lesions are detected from the age of 20 peaking at about 40-50 years. Breast cancer is seen in increasing frequency after menopause.

Breast Examination

The size of the breast may make it difficult to detect lumps by self breast examination without learning the proper technique. Begin by inspecting one's breast standing in front of a mirror with the hands pressed against the hips. The nipple, areola and overlying skin are inspected for smoothness and abnormal discharges. Later this is repeated with the hands raised above the head which allows one to notice abnormalities.

When one arm is raised, the palm of the other hand can be used to examine the opposite breast feeling systematically. Finally the nipples should be expressed to determine if there is a discharge. The manoeuver is repeated on the opposite breast.

Table 16.1 Steps in Self Breast Examination

Step	Manoeuver	What to look for
1.	Look at both breasts in mirror with shoulder straight and hands on hip	Are breasts symmetrical in shape and size Any swellings Skin contour smooth /inflamed No puckering of skin No discharge from breast (clear fluid, yellow or blood)
2.	Raise arms placing them behind the neck and look for the same as in (1)	May squeeze nipples to look for discharge, look for symmetry (normal)
3.	Lie down on bed, and with the right hand begin to feel left breast systematically. Use the pad of the fingers keeping fingers flat. The aim is to feel the entire breast including the breast tail extending into the arm pit. Begin with a circular motion from nipple and move out or perform a up and down motion. Repeat the procedure on the right breast using the left hand. To feel the deeper part of the breast one needs to exert some pressure . You should be able to appreciate the chest wall and overlying muscles	Lumps and nodularity
4.	Repeat step 3 sitting or during bath when the skin is wet and smooth.	Feeling texture of breast is better appreciated

What does one look for?

This is a common question a woman may ask. Basically, look for asymmetry, lumps in the breast tissue and enlarged glands in the armpit. Examine for changes in contour of skin and changes in nipple shape and nipple discharge. Bloody nipple discharge and puckering of the skin (like that of orange skin) require medical attention. Skin may be swollen and tender because of infection (mastitis). Ulcers are late manifestation of malignancy.

When a doctor performs the breast examination, a verbal consent is obtained and all her upper garments up to the waist have to be removed. A chaperone is in attendance. The examination is done standing, sitting and lying down. The sitting position permits ease of examination of the neck and armpit for detection of swellings due to enlarged lymph nodes. When the patient lies down, a pillow placed between the shoulder blades with the right arm raised above the head would make deeper examination of the right breast thorough. The steps explained in Table 16.1 would be followed. The examination of the left breast then follows with the respective arm raised.

Looking for asymmetry may require the patient to raise the head in a standing position, bending forward with raised arms. This would throw the breasts forward and hang freely.

Having inspected and examined the breasts examination of lymph nodes in the armpit (axilla) and neck, behind the collar bones are essential for a complete evaluation. The lymphatic system of the breast was discussed above. The neck nodes are best felt with the doctor standing behind the patient and the axillary lymph nodes are better felt with the corresponding elbow slightly raised.

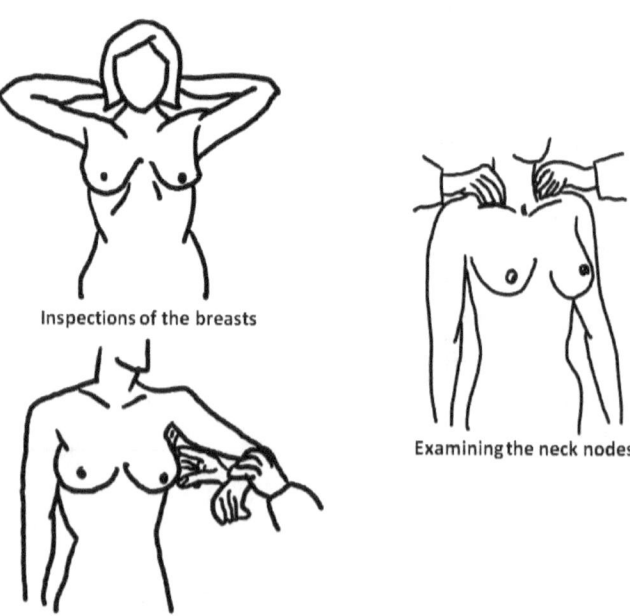

Inspections of the breasts

Examining the neck nodes

Feeling for the nodes in the armpit

Fig. 16.3: Examining the Lymph Nodes

Knowing the difference between normal and abnormal findings

The breasts are endocrine glands responding to female hormones. Their primary function is to be able to lactate and feed the young from birth. Changes in growth are noticed from puberty and enlargement is expected with pregnancy. As menopause sets in, estrogen depletion will cause the breast tissue to become smaller and support is weak resulting is sagging.

Breast tenderness and discomfort is felt in early pregnancy. Breasts enlarge under the influence of pregnancy hormones with little buds lining the areola increasing in number with advancing pregnancy. The colour of the nipple darkens with time in pregnancy. Slight watery discharge is normal during pregnancy. Milky discharge is present after the birth of the child and not when a woman is not pregnant. Should milk be expressed in non-pregnant state there could be over-activity of the brain producing the hormone, prolactin?

When the patient is not pregnant, she may notice some changes in the breast throughout the menstrual cycle with discomfort becoming more prominent before menstruation. The breasts will invariably involute after menopause.

Every symptom or sign a patient has must be taken seriously so as not to miss a diagnosis of cancer, though a majority of symptoms noticed before menopause are not due to breast cancer. Compassionate and realistic approach will be kinder to the woman with symptoms, as most women's fear of cancer is real and the attending health provider, be it a nurse or doctor needs to be thorough in evaluation. The three tools commonly used in diagnosis of cancer of the breast are mammogram, breast ultrasound and fine need aspiration (FNA), a small surgical procedure. These investigations should be done only if they are indicated. There are local guidelines for medical personal to follow in utilizing these investigations and women should have access to these guidelines written 'plain language'. Reassurance in menopausal women having symptoms especially if they have been on hormone therapy for a long period should only be given after thoroughly eliciting vital history, performance of a complete physical examination and doing relevant tests.

Benign Breast Disease

Benign disease refers to conditions that are not cancerous. In dedicated breast screening centres, perhaps about 85% of all breast disease is benign. Breast pain is not common in breast cancer, presenting in less than 10 % of patients. The subsequent discussion on benign breast disease contains technical terms but are worthy of note. Much benign disease may not be frequently seen in the menopausal age but are mentioned for completeness sake.

Benign disease of the breast could be categorized according to age groups and relate to development of breast tissues.

i. Adolescence

During the adolescent years breast tissues grow rapidly differentiating into specialised cells under the influence of female hormones. One form of abnormal growth that has been described is HYPERTROPHY because of excessive growth, which is not of great clinical significance. Another condition is FIBROADENOMA or 'breast mice'. Fibroadenoma is a benign disease related to disorderly growth of tissues often presenting in women between 15-25 years of age. Fibroadenoma rarely is diagnosed after 35 years. The patient may have a single solitary tumour or several of them measuring about 3 cm in diameter each. Most women would request surgical removal though FNAC would be a better option to make a diagnosis.

ii. Reproductive age

Two complaints in this age group (15-50 years):

a) Mastalgia
b) Nodularity

Mastalgia refers to breast pain. Nodularity refers to a feeling of lumpiness in the breast without the ability to definitely identify a specific lump. Nearly 50% of medical consults for breast problems relate to these two complaints. Although most women are fearful of breast cancer, it would be reassuring to know that less than 10% of breast cancer cases have breast pain as a symptom. There are variety of causes for breast pain and an equal number of treatment options. Thorough questioning about relationship of symptom to menstrual cycle should be elicited. Relieving and aggravating factors should also be enquired into.

The most common form of breast pain that is associated with the female hormone fluctuation during menstruation is called CYCLICAL MASTALGIA. Pain is felt in both breasts and often feels worse a few days before the onset of menstrual flow. Nodularity of the breast is also obvious during this time. Pain may take the form of heaviness or increased sensitivity. Patients who are worried and fearful of cancer when MASTALGIA is severe and incapacitating lasting a week, they can be assured that it is most probably a benign disease.

When 'breast pain' is not related to the menstrual cycle, occurs only in one breast or first noticed just before or after menopause, further evaluation with standard tests are required. In this situation nodularity is uncommon or be 'fleeting' in nature. There may be a lack of the smooth feel of the overlying skin, called 'puckering'.

Breast pain management is not due to breast cancer in most instances and reassurance is all that is required after complete evaluation. Simple measures include advice on changing the size of brassieres if they are ill-fitting should be given. Explanation on value of diet modification is warranted. Avoiding coffee, chocolate and Cola will decrease the stimulatory effects caffeine had on the breast. Analgesics (pain killers) and minor tranquillizers are reserved for a few women who do not respond to measures mentioned. Hormones and medication are final resorts. Commonly used drugs are DANAZOL, progestogen and bromocriptine.

Table 16.2 Characteristics of Breast Pain

Features	Cyclical Breast Pain	Non-cyclical Breast Pain
Usual age	>30 years	>40 years
Area of breast affected	Both Breasts All over the breast	One Breast (unilateral) Usually over a specific area
Relation to menstruation	Yes	No
Occurring after menopause	Rare	About 12%
Successful treatment with hormones	>80%	<40%

iii. Menopausal age

As menopause approaches, breast tissue shrinks or involutes in an organized way in response to estrogen decline. If the involution process is not organised, fibrous tissue may shrink leaving behind some glandular tissue which continue to be functional. As these glandular tissue are in communication with ducts, they get 'strangulated' resulting in CYST FORMATION. As they are sited at a particular area of the breast they may mimic a tumor.

In treating patients with breast cyst, ultrasonography is very helpful. However, cysts less that 3-5 mm in diameter will not be well imaged. In such instances mammogram is preferred. Fine needle aspiration (FNA) of the cyst would provide confirmatory evidence of thee nature of the cyst.

As we conclude this discussion on benign changes that can occur at various stages of the woman's life, we should also be mindful of the other organs that lie behind the breast which may be afflicted by disease, symptoms of which may be thought to be arising from the breast. Muscles, tendons and the rib cage may the origin of pain related to infections, trauma and tumor. Diseases of the pleura, lungs and even heart disease may be needed to be excluded when breast pain is reported.

Some of the uncommon benign diseases that are seen affecting the breast are listed in Table 16.4.

Table 16.3: Benign Diseases of the Breast

Condition	Characteristics
Supernumerary Breast Tissue (these are extra 'breasts' that appear as small lumps)	These are breast tissue with areola and nipple but no duct is present leading to obstruction Found in side of the chest, axilla and other parts of body
Inflammation (infection manifested by localized pain and even fever)	Mastitis—no mass is felt
	Granulomatous mastitis—can be due to foreign material, autoimmune disorder or tuberculosis
Foreign Body Reaction (foreign body are artificial material implanted in breasts)	Silicone, paraffin can cause reaction May be seen after breast re-construction or breast augmentation
Mammary duct ectasia	Nipple discharge and pain may be present
Fat necrosis (this refers to 'self destruction ' of fat cells in the breasts)	Can follow surgery on the breast or trauma May mimic tumor as ill defined speculated image on mammogram
Fibrocystic disease of breast (manifests as lumps in breasts and can cause pain especially during menstruation)	Occurs between 20-50 years Often bilateral and multifocal Breast pain and tenderness common symptoms Due to hormonal imbalance
Breast cysts (most often detected at mammogram and ultrasound examination of breasts)	Occurs between 30-50 years Filled with clear fluid Often ovoid in shape Ultrasound imaging is warranted Fine needle aspiration FNAC may be indicated

Discharge from the Nipple

Clear fluid and milk can discharge from the nipple. Many of such discharges are not sinister and are usually benign. Only 2 % of breast cancer patients present with abnormal nipple discharge.

The structure and functions of the breast has been elaborated in the earlier section of this chapter. Both hormones and drugs can affect breast function. Patients who have been taking hormonal contraceptives and psychotropic drugs (for severe depression and schizophrenia) may discharge milk from the nipples, referred to as GALACTORRHOEA. A similar condition can be seen in women with a small benign tumor of the pituitary gland called PROLACTINOMA where high levels of the hormone PROLACTIN are detected in the blood.

Sexual stimulation and regular self expression of the breasts can produce secretions; these are considered normal.

If the abnormal discharge is confined to a single breast and is bloody or mixed with serous fluid, a consultation is required to determine the underlying cause. Pus discharge is not normal and is strongly suggestive of bacterial infection. If a lump or nodule is present with nipple discharge further tests have to be done with urgency. There is a need to exclude either a papilloma or cancer of the breast. Women above the age of 50 need closer scrutiny with mammogram, ultrasound scanning and aspiration of cells and fluid with a fine needle (FNAC). DUCTAL ECTASIA is a benign disease but may present with the above symptoms.

Breast Cancer: Figures and Risks Summarised

Breast cancer is now considered a public health problem. The World Health Organization (WHO) estimates that breast cancer incidence will increase by 14.5% due to increase in life expectancy in women coupled with environmental and lifestyle changes. Improvement in survival of breast cancer victim can be envisaged with effective screening programs and early detection of the disease.

In the US about 230000 women are diagnosed each year. The rates of cancer of the breast showed a decreasing trend, dropping by 7% from 2002-2003 because of a marked decline in use of hormone therapy following a Women's Health Initiative findings published in 2002. The research findings showed a small but noticeable link of estrogen-progestogen hormone therapy to both breast cancer and heart disease.

The WHO estimated that over half a million women died of breast cancer in 2004 and that this could have been markedly reduced through education and breast screening programs. If all women lived to 70 (US life time risk) 1:8 women would have developed breast cancer. Developed countries (Americas, UK, Australia, and New Zealand) had higher rates of newly diagnosed breast cancer but survival rates are poorer in developing countries because of late detection and poor screening programs.

Inadequate awareness programs on breast cancer and cultural factors are common in women not coming forward for screening. Poor access to mammograms is an issue in countries with poor resources and self breast examination is not found to be an effective tool in early detection of the disease. Smoking is more common in developed countries and has been associated with breast cancer prevalence.

The cause of breast cancer is not known although much research is in progress in understanding the development of the cancer. Genetic and environmental factors are implicated. Some of the known risk factors are discussed below.

a. Racial Factors

Caucasian women and African-American under 40 years have a slightly higher risk of developing breast cancer than Asian women.

b. Family History

If a first degree relative (sister or mother) has had cancer of the breast, there is an increased risk for the woman. The risk is even higher if the relative had developed the disease before menopause. A doubling of risk is seen with one relative affected and this increases five fold if two such relatives are affected.

Genetic linkage is apparent in breast cancer. Two familial breast cancer genes are known to be associated with breast cancer viz. BRCA1 or BRCA2. The risk is >80% if there are genetic alterations to these genes. Fortunately only about 2% of breast cancers are associated with these gene mutations.

A family history of cancer of the ovaries and uterus places the woman at a higher risk.

Although most benign conditions are not associated with breast cancer some abnormal lesions like atypical hyperplasia (lobular or ductal) or lobular carcinoma in situ have a 4 times higher risk.

Age

More than 75% of women diagnosed with breast cancer are above the age of 50 years with 50% being more than 65 years of age.

c. History of cancer

If one breast is involved there is a 7-10 times higher risk of the other breast being involved.

d. Parity and childbirth

Women who have not borne children have a higher rate of breast cancer. The risk is also higher if pregnancy is deferred to a later age (after 35 years). A reduction from 6.3/100 to 2.7/100 cumulative cases of breast cancer is extrapolated in one study where women increased parity from 2.7 to 6.5 and breast feed longer from 8 months to 24 months.

Menarche and Menstrual cycles

Early menarche before 12 years and late menopause after 55 means these women have many more menstrual cycles. An increased risk seen in these women may be related to longer duration of estrogen stimulation. Pregnancy and breast feeding clearly have protective effect in women.

e. Hormones

The role of hormones will be discussed under the relevant chapter. There is no good evidence to advice against the use of oral hormonal contraceptives in the reproductive age group.

f. Diet

There is a small correlation between breast cancers and taking fatty food, red meat and food that contains fine sugar. Alcohol and obesity are other risk factors. A 1.5 times higher risk is noted in women who take 2-5 drinks daily.

Some controversy reigns on the association of hormonal birth control pills as breast cancer. While some studies have suggested that women who on hormonal birth control pills have a very slight increased risk of developing breast cancer others refute this. The reported risk, however, disappears after stopping them for 10 years or more. More research is being done before a clear picture emerges.

g. Irradiation

Exposure to high dose radiation increases the risk.

Breast Cancer and Hormone Therapy

The Women's Health Intiative study demonstrated an increase of breast cancer when a combination of estrogen and progesterone hormone regime was prescribed (unadjusted risk ratio of 1.26 over 5.2 years). Women at greatest risk were those who had been on this combination for over 10 years of treatment. Only a slight increase in risk was seen in those who took the hormone combination for less than 5 years. Women who had taken only estrogen as they had had hysterectomy done were better off and did not show a similar pattern.

Mammograms appear to be affected when medical hormone therapy is taken with some differences between taking combined hormone therapy and estrogen only regime. This evidence was derived form the PEPI trial (Postmenopausal Estrogen/Progestin Interventions). Increased breast density was seen in those on estrogen with micronized progestogen (16.4%)which was higher than those with estrogen only (16.4% vs, 3.5%). Increasing breast density appears to be associated with increases in breast cancer. Women will discuss with their doctor on implications of breast density and breast cancer risk as individual risk factors need to be considered before making generalizations from the information given. Current guidelines will dictate how hormones must be prescribed.

Conclusion

Having a risk factor does not mean the woman would definitely develop breast cancer. More than 75% of women who develop breast cancer do not have a risk factor. Women who have high risk should regularly perform self breast examination and enter a screening program at an earlier age than those without risk factors. Although controversial, presence of a benign disorder does not place the woman under 'risk' category. Hormone therapy is not a good option in women who have a risk of developing breast cancer. Oral hormone contraceptives are permitted in the reproductive age this is the most acceptable form of contraception. Breast feeding plays a protective role and should be encouraged.

Reference:

Collaborative Group on Hormonal Factors in Breast Cancer Breast cancer and breastfeeding: collaborative reanalysis of individual data from 47 epidemiological studies in 30 countries, including 50302 women with breast cancer and 96973 women without the disease. Lancet 2002; 360; 9328; 187-

CHAPTER 17

CANCER OF THE BREAST—
THE SCARE

In the 1970s cancer of the breast was termed 'THE FOREMOST CANCER'. It still is! In the Netherlands it accounts for 21% of female deaths. Worldwide, it remains the commonest cancer in women. Treatment for breast cancer has undergone tremendous changes over the last three decades ranging from radical surgery to more conservative 'breast saving' approaches with radiation and chemotherapy. Reconstructive surgery is now becoming important component of primary surgical treatment.

The discussion that follows cannot be an elaborate discourse on cancer of the breast. Suffice to state that there appears to be two groups of women with breast cancer, one below 50 years and another group beyond 50 years. On-going research will shed more light in the years to come how genetic profiling and epidemiologic factors contribute to the development of cancers in these two groups of women.

Preventive strategies like screening for breast cancer will help detect early disease so that survival after appropriate treatment will be longer. Controversies reign on the value of self breast examination as to whether it is worthwhile a method in detecting disease. The link between estrogen hormone therapy and the occurrence of invasive breast cancer has been discussed. Physicians need to be well versed with current thoughts on long term use of estrogen and progestogen hormone therapy and be able to explain the meaning of terms like 'RELATIVE RISK' when counselling women on hormone therapy. Women will continue to avail information on consensus views on best practice in screening for breast cancers and latest views on treatment of invasive breast cancer and the use of hormone therapy through social media and lay press.

(i) Cardiovascular disease

In the chapter on heart and blood vessels, we related three disease states that women encounter in the menopausal years i.e cardiovascular disease, osteoporosis and breast cancer. Deaths due to coronary heart disease and strokes occur more frequently compared to deaths following complications of osteoporosis and breast cancer. In developed countries there are more breast cancer survivors now because of detection of early stage of breast cancer following effective screening for breast cancer.

In Australia cardiovascular disease is the leading cause of death coronary heart disease accounting for 16.6% and strokes accounting for 10% of all deaths. Breast cancer deaths are estimated to be 4% of total deaths (AIHW, 2006 statistics).

These facts need to be highlighted when counselling women in the older age group.

(ii) Risk Factors for Breast Cancer

Is breast cancer predictable or preventable? Although this question is difficult to answer one needs to determine if the known risk factors help us to educate women in methods to screen for the disease. Some women are inevitably more prone to develop breast cancer even in the absence of known risk factors (listed in Table 17.1).

The risk factors for women developing breast cancer are similar in the East and West. These are highlighted in chapter 17. Exposure to female hormones produced within the body (endogenous), genetic factors, and diet with certain lifestyles have been mentioned. Clearly various environmental factors will impact on these risk factors in some. It is now clear that women who have been breastfeeding and consume diets high in tofu and other soy proteins are less likely to develop breast cancer. On the other hand, those who have a longer period of exposure to endogenous hormones like early onset of menstruation (menarche) and late menopause are more prone. Obesity is related to diet and genetic factors. Smoking and obesity are not only linked to breast cancer but also to cardiovascular disease and lung disease.

Table17.1 Risk Factors for Breast Cancer

Factor	Comment
Gender	Women have 100 X higher risk than men
Age	Risk increase with age 2/3 women with invasive cancer are >55 years
Genetic predisposition	5-10% Mutations of gene (BRCA1, BRCA 2) have 80% risk
Family History	Although 80% of women with cancer have no family history, those with a family history (mother or sister) carry higher risk
Personal history	Risk of cancer on the contralateral breast is higher
Lobular carcinoma in-situ	Though not cancerous, carry higher risk, need close follow-up
Menstrual pattern	Those with menarche<12 and menopause >55 (endogenous hormone)

(iii) Screening for breast cancer

Prevention is better than cure, so goes the dictum. This statement is so true for breast cancer. It is also generally true that screening methods do not prevent disease but contribute to early diagnosis and better prognosis. The breasts are easily accessible for examination unlike many other organs of the body. Screening methods like self breast examination, ultrasonography and mammogram are useful because of this fact.

Although all women should be screened for breast cancer after the age of 50 years, those with risk factors should be more vigilant in coming forth to avail themselves for screening.

Self breast examination for abnormalities in the skin texture and lumps is by far the cheapest of the existing screening tools. Many simple pamphlets are available that teaches self breast examination. Breast self examination ought to be done in a systematic manner. Abnormal discharge from the breast nipple and any bloody discharge should be evaluated immediately.

There has been much criticism about the value of breast examination (both by physicians and patient alike) as it has not been found to be a sensitive tool for detecting tumors. Although this is true, in developing countries, self breast examination continues to be taught as it increases client awareness and is value for health education. In many institutes, WELL WOMEN clinics have been established to provide care for women to maintain a healthy life. Healty women should utilize this amenities and come forward for screening especially when they attain the age of 50 years. At the same sitting they should also have pap smears done (if they have not had one in the preceding 2-3 years) and seek general advice on menopause. Large scale national screening programs like the 'DOM-project' in Utrecht, Netherlands (started in 1974) aimed at screening women aged 50-74 years has appealed to most except for 2% of the population.

a. Mammogram

The mammogram has come into vogue over the last 30 years as an effective screening tool. It involves taking radiographs of both the breasts and can detect a tumor long before it can be felt as 'lump'. Current guidelines suggest routine mammogram for women beyond 50 years. Only women with high risk for breast cancer are recommended for mammogram below 50 years. The level of radiation is low.

During a mammnogram a female radiologist will assist in placing one breast at a time on a plastic plate. A second piece of plastic plate will be placed on top for a few seconds. Some pressure is applied so as to flatten the breast. This may cause some discomfort. Films are then taken and the procedure repeated on the other breast. The procedure takes about 20-25 minutes.

The radiographs will be immediately developed and reported by the radiologist. At times it is difficult to say if a 'shadow' seen is cancerous. An ultrasound or more tests (biopsy) may be required.

b. Ultrasound examination of the breast

The ultrasound machine uses high frequency sounds though a small transducer. The latter is placed on the breast after application of a lubricant. Images are seen on a monitor. This procedure is not painful and no radiation is used (only sound waves).

c. Fine Needle Biopsy

Should a lump be detected the radiologist would perform a fine needle biopsy (FNAC) after a local anaesthesia is administered to the area over the breast. The needle is fine and the method is a rapid means of taking tissue from the breast lump. Most times an ultrasound guide is used. Cells aspirated after passing the needle into the tissues are aspirated and placed on a glass slide, stained and examined under a microscope to detect cancer cells.

(iv) Facts and Figures

Although estrogen (hormone) therapy is beneficial for women who suffer from hot flashes, night sweats and vaginal dryness after the menopause, its association with increase in breast cancer has caused both scepticism and alarm to both women and the medical fraternity for its prolonged use. The general public often access information on the risks of hormone therapy from the media. Some of this information may be difficult to interpret or understand in view of the use of statistical information like risk ratios and mean values. In order to evaluate data derived fro scientific research, care givers need to be consulted as to risks and benefits.

Historically two scientific trials (between 1998-2002) drew the medical fraternity to improved understanding of the impact of hormones in women during the menopause viz. HERS and WHI studies. In 2002, the increase risk of breast cancer with use of estrogen/progesterone with an added risk for coronary heart disease, stroke and pulmonary embolism from the WHI study enabled review and re-drawing of guidelines in use of hormone therapy. Similarly, the use of estrogen only hormone was cautioned after the results of the WHI showed that there was an increased risk for stroke and pulmonary embolism (blot clot in the lungs). The decline in use of hormone therapy was noticeable in the US after these results were disclosed. Since then numerous reports have been released on selective use of hormones.

The WHI steering committee (2004) released the relative risks of hormone therapy with lowest seen in reduction of hip fractures (0.61 highest in stroke (1.39). The North American Menopause Society (2010) summarise the following in use of hormone therapy:

- All women should be counselled about risks and benefits
- Hormones are best in treating women with moderate and severe vasomotor (hot flashes) symptoms
- The lowest effective dose of hormones should be prescribed and that too not longer than 3-5 years
- The hormones should not be initiated in women >60 years of age

The US Preventive Health Service Task Force takes a rather extreme view and states that hormone therapy should not be for routine use in those with chronic postmenopausal women. This would have implications when estrogen is prescribed to prevent osteoporosis.

Table 17.2 Summary of Guidelines for Medical Hormone Therapy in USA

American College of Obstetrics and Gynecology 2002	Encourage prior counselling of women about risks and benefits State risk reduction, diet, exercise, weight management, smoking cessation and alcohol reduction Lowest dose of effective hormone dose for shortest duration
North American Menopause Society 2008 & 2010	Counsel women about risks and benefits Treat women with moderate and severe vasomotor symptoms or to prevent risk of fracture (osteoporosis) in some high risk women Not to treat for longer than 3-5 years with lowest effective dose Should not be prescribed for women>60 years
US Preventive Health Services Task Force 2005	Categorically against use of medical hormone therapy for prevention of chronic disorders in postmenopausal women

Breast cancer with the use of medical hormone therapy is always of great concern and women need to be aware of the risks involved. It is now clear that prolonged use increases the risk with an absolute increase seen in some diseases after 3-5 years of continuous use. This is the reason that current guidelines do not recommend hormone use beyond this duration. (Table 17.1). The risk is compounded with initiation of both progestogen with estrogen (combined therapy) as opposed to estrogen therapy alone. Women who smoke and consume alcohol beyond social drinking while on hormone therapy almost double the known risk of developing breast cancer. Current guidelines do not recommend use of medical combined hormone therapy after 60 years of age.

a. What is relative risk

Relative risk illustrates the likelihood of developing the disease in a group of people who are exposed to the disease as compared to a group who are not exposed (i.e those who are taking hormones against those who do not).

Relative Risk (RR) = <u>No. of women taking hormones</u>
No. of women not taking hormones

If RR =1, the incidence in the exposed group of women (i.e those taking hormones) and non-exposed are the same i.e there is no increased risk. If the RR=1.5, then the exposed group have a 50% more likely risk of developing the disease. If the RR=0.4, then the exposed is 40% less likely to develop the disease.

b. Criticism directed to clinical study

In analysing the data, several factors are considered about people in the study groups so as to make the findings valid. The use of estrogen alone or in combination with progestogen, the route of administration (oral, applied to skin, inserted in the vagina etc), the age when it was intiated (how soon after menopause), the duration of treatment (years of therapy) and the presence of risk factors (age, obesity, underlying hypertension, hyperlipidemia, smoking, alcohol consumption, life style) need to be factored in. Epidemiological studies often factor these issues in interpretation but it may not be easy to take into consideration all the factors.

Some women are genetically prone to develop some chronic diseases and these are not easy to exclude when people from the general population are selected for the study. Hence a perfect experiment is often not possible.

Parkin DM (British Journal of Cancer 2011) estimated that about 3% (1530 cases) of breast cancers in the United Kingdom were directly linked to hormone therapy. In about 75% of those women were taking a combination of estrogen and progestogen.

Table 17.3 Relative risk of invasive breast cancer in hormone and non-hormone users (Source: UK Cancer Research)

Use of hormone	Relative Risk
Never used	1.00
Currently using	1.66
Currently using estrogen only	1.30
Currently using estrogen-progestogen	2.00
Currently using Tibolone (a different type of hormone)	1.45
Had had used in the past	1.01
Last used less than 5 years previously	1.04
Last used 5-9 years previously	1.01
Last used more than 10 years previosly	0.90

A family history of breast cancer is related to genetic predisposition but the overall incidence is low. These rare familial cancer are shown below.

Table 17.4 Rare Cancers seen in families

Gene	Syndrome	Cancers associated with gene
BRCA1	Breast/ovarian predisposition	Breast, ovary, bowel, prostate
BRCA2	Breast/ovarian predisposition	Breast, ovary, bowel, prostate, pancreas
PTEN	Cowden's syndrome	Breast, thyroid, gut
STK11/LKB1	Peutz-Jeghers Syndrome	Breast, ovary, gut, pancreas

Source: Sunday People 19 May 2013

Angeline Jolie has the BRCA1 gene that has a 87% risk of breast cancer and 50% risk of ovarian cancer in the long run. By taking the bold move to have bilateral mastectomy this film actor has reduced her risk of breast cancer to less than 5%.

Being Overweight and Having a Dense Breast

The breast constitutes of fat and tissues referred to as connective tissue (which support the breast and epithelial tissue. When the amount of fat is less in quantity we call it less dense. Apparently when the density of the breast is high (i.e less proportion of fat) there is a five times higher risk of breast cancer (McCormack VA, Cancer Epidemiology Biomarkers Prev 2006; 15:1159-69)

Overweight and breast cancer appear to have some relationship and strategies to reduce body weight has an overall positive effect. Usually one would consider both height of the woman and her weight in Kg and work out the body mass index. Should the BMI be more than 25-29.9 she is overweight and when the BMI >30 she is obese. The overweight postmenopausal women have a 10-20% increased risk of breast cancer while this figure increases to 30 time higher in obese postmenopausal women.

Both alcohol and smoking have been implicated in increases of breast cancer risk. Excess alcohol has been shown to be linked but the association with smoking is debatable. If women began smoking before 20 years of age perhaps there may be at a higher risk but there is need for more data to support this statement.

Is Hormone Therapy Safe for Menopausal symptoms?

The answer to this question will continue to be debated and its use will be based on benefit derived and risks of individual patient. More than 20 research studies have been done since the 1970s and the results vary according to the body system. Hormones are effective in preventing osteoporosis. Certainly it is the best medication to relieve bothersome hot flashes and vaginal dryness. As the WHI and the Million Women study show an increased risk for breast cancer more stringent rules are in place for its use e.g using the lowest does and for the shortest duration.

Colditz's research group studied 367187 person-years who were menopausal registered nurses (the Nurse's Health Study) and reported these figures some twenty years ago

Current users had high RR (1.30 in estrogen only and 2.0 in combined estrogen-progestogen groups). Alcohol consumption was an associated factor. An interesting information from sub-analysis of the data indicated that age at last time estrogen was taken and the dose of hormone also had an effect on the RR. The RR improved from 0.99 to 1.09 one year after cessation of estrogen. After a lapse of 10 years (of not taking estrogen) the RR was 0.90.

To help understand the risks current information on association of medical hormone therapy and breast cancer should be sought from reliable sources and shared with menopausal women. The following information is worthy of repetition:

There is a small increase in breast cancer incidence if a woman is on medial hormone therapy (estrogen and progestogen combination having a higher risk than estrogen alone). This risk increases when the hormone therapy is taken for long durations. However, the risk of developing breast cancer is the same as the non-users if they have been off the hormones for at least five years. Age, duration of use and if the hormone is estrogen-only or a combination (estrogen + progestogen) appear to impact on the incidence of breast cancer apart from other factors mentioned above including life style.

Table 17.5 Risk of Breast Cancer by age, use, non-use and duration of hormone use

Use of Hormone Therapy (HT)	Breast Cancer Risk 50-59 years	Breast Cancer Risk 60-69 years
No Hormone Therapy	10/1000	15/1000
Estrogen Only HT for 5 years	Extra 2/1000	3/1000
Estrogen-Progestogen HT for 5 years	Extra 6/1000	9/1000
No Hormone Therapy (10 year period)	20/1000	30/1000
Estrogen only HT for 10 years	Extra 6/1000	Extra 9/1000
Estrogen—Progestogen HT for 10 years	24/1000	Extra 36/1000

Source: http://www.patient.co.uk/health/menopause-and-hrt

Alternatives to conventional hormone therapy

With the release of new data on the increased risk of breast cancer with longer duration of hormone therapy especially the combined form (estrogen and progestogen) there has been a reported decline in total use over the last decade. However, women have been resorting to alternative medication including bio-identical prescriptions thinking it would be safer as most are derived from plant.

Common preparations are black cohosh, red clover, dong quai, evening primrose oil, ginseng, and kava. The 'Clinical Knowledge Summaries' report does not recommend the use of complementary therapies for the following reasons:

- The preparation and quality of each varies
- Long term safety especially on the lining of the uterus (endometrium) and breast has not be clearly established
- The efficacy needs to be established by conventional methods of testing
- Some (black cohosh, red clover and ginseng) have effects like that of estrogen and may not be suitable (for those with or prone to develop breast cancer)

- Serious side effects have been reported (e.g. liver damage seen in kava and black cohosh; anticoagulant effect seen in red clover and dong quai as they contain coumarins)

Source: Royal College of Obstetricians and Gynecologists. Alternatives to HRT for management of symptoms of the menopause (Scientific Impact Paper 6) Sept 2006, retrieved 20th May 2013

Conclusions

Breast cancer is the commonest malignancy among women. A small proportion of women carry mutated genes that increases the chances of development of breast cancer markedly. A large number of women who eventually develop the cancer may not have risk factors. However, in those who have an identifiable risk factor should be screened for the disease. Hormone therapy which consists of estrogen alone (in those who have had hysterectomy) and combined (estrogen and progesterone) is effective for treatment of vasomotor symptoms (palpitations, hot flashes and night sweats) and also for urogenital problems (atrophic vaginitis and painful intercourse).

Hormones should not be prescribed solely to protect against bone loss. Short term use with the minimal dose necessary for symptom relief will not increase the risk of breast cancer in women who are not at risk. However, long term use especially beyond five years and particularly with the combined hormones has been associated with an increase in the absolute number of breast cancer when compared to 'non-users'. Women should consult physicians and also be monitored periodically when hormones are are used in indicated cases. Bio-identical hormones cannot be recommended as 'safe alternatives' till more robust data is available.

References

1. Cancer Research United Kingdom
2. Cancer advice http://www.canceradvice.co.uk/breast-cancer/
3. http://www.cancerresearchuk.org/cancer-info/cancerstats/types/breast/riskfactors/breast-cancer-risk-factors (retrieved 19 May 2013)

CHAPTER 18

CANCER OF THE UTERUS—
What you should know?

Cancer of the uterus basically constitutes that which affects the cervix (carcinoma of the cervix) and endometrial cancer (affecting the inner lining of the uterine cavity). Knowledge about the genesis of both these tumors has increased markedly over the years. Most patients who develop cancer of the cervix are younger (below 50 years) and currently the human papilloma virus is implicated. Cancer of the endometrium is often seen in the older age group, usually well after menopause though a small proportion of women develop it when they are younger.

The Uterus

The womb is referred to as the uterus. This pear shaped organ of the female genital tract is situated in the pelvis with the urinary bladder lying in front and the rectum, behind. The uterus has much larger bulky muscular portion called the corpus which has the endometrium lining the uterine cavity. The lower narrower portion, the cervix opens into the vagina establishing continuity between the uterine cavity and the vagina. Any abnormal bleeding in the menopause age is hence manifested as bleeding per vaginum. This is one of the reasons practitioners perform a vaginal examination whenever women in the menopause age complain of abnormal bleeding.

The cervix is accessible (because of its location) through a vaginal speculum facilitating taking of pap smear and also enabling the passage of devices into the uterine cavity to obtain specimens (endometrial biopsy) should the patient have abnormal bleeding from the uterine cavity.

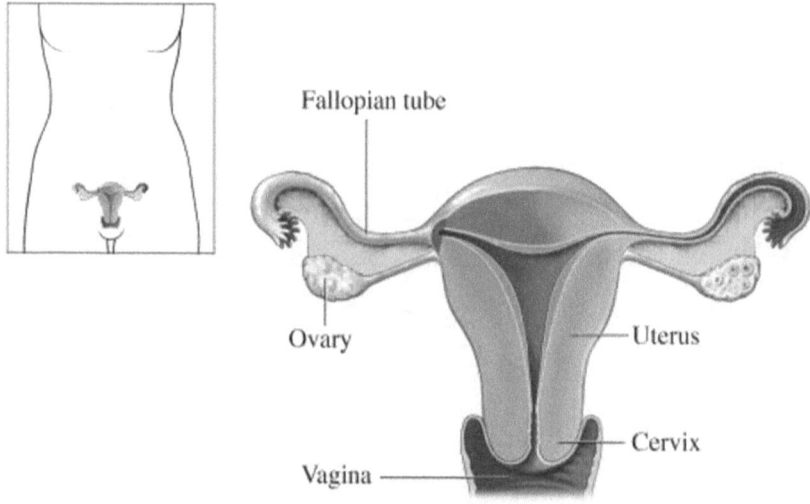

Figure 18.1 Diagram of Uterus (front view)

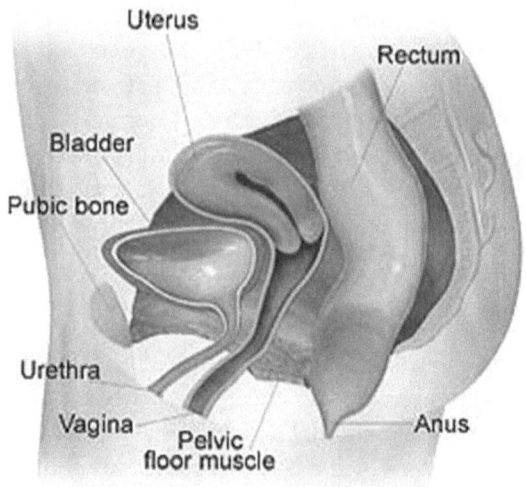

Figure 18.1 Diagram of Pelvic Organs (Front and Side Views)

Although the lining of the uterus (endometrium) becomes very thin after menopause because estrogen levels from the ovaries decline rapidly small amounts of a different type of estrogen (estrone) are derived from 'tiny amounts of male hormone, androgen' found in the ageing ovary and adrenal glands. This transformation from androgen to estrone occurs mainly in the fat cells of the body. It is possible that cumulative amounts of estrone influence the endometrium to develop tumors in the endometrium. This explanation may apply to the development of endometrial cancer.

CANCER OF THE UTERUS

Two common types of cancers of the uterus are cervical cancer and uterine (endometrial) cancer. Cervical cancer occurs in younger women especially between 35-50 years. Sexual promiscuity and multiple sexual partners lead to increased risk of genital infections especially human papilloma virus infection (HPV) which are implicated in cancer of the cervix.

Uterine cancer is seen in older women and most are seen in the menopausal years of age.

CANCER OF THE CERVIX

The incidence of cancer of the cervix varies throughout the world with higher mortality occurring in developing countries. The main types of cervical cancers are SQUAMOUS CELL CARCINOMA and ADENOCARCINOMA OF THE CERVIX. Although more than 100 types of HPV are known about 40 can be passed to the woman during sexual intercourse. Genital warts is caused by a similar virus but does not cause cervical cancer.

It is estimated that half a million women worldwide die of cancer of the cervix annually. Eighty to eighty-five percent are from the developing world where women are socially disadvantaged, poor, illiterate and have no access to healthcare. As shown in Fig.18.2 the African, Latin American and some Asian countries are worst affected. The risk factors for developing cervical cancer after HPV infection are shown below.

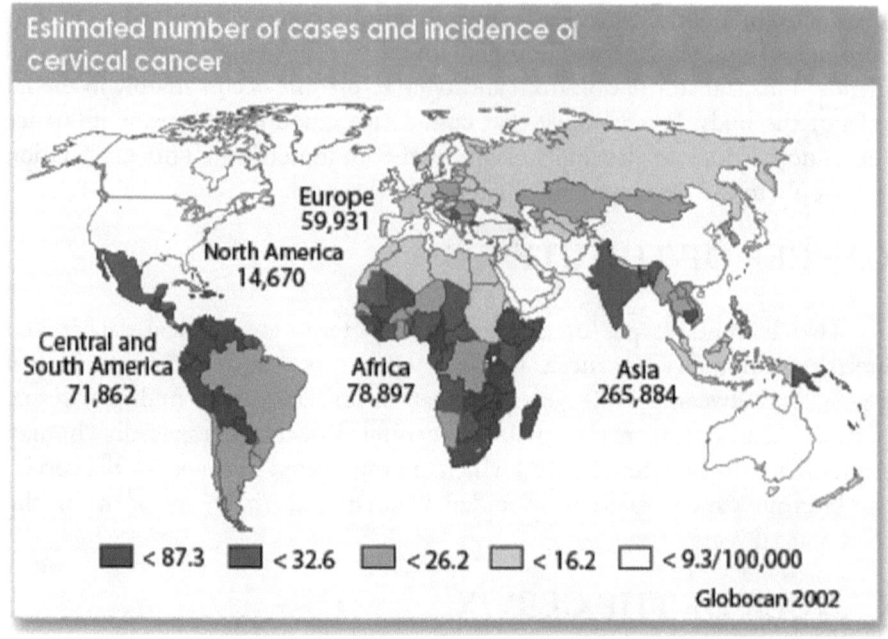

Figure 18.2 Cervical Cancer Worldwide

Source: RHO Cervical Cancer, Globocan 2002.

Risk Factors for developing cervical cancer after HPV infection

- Early age at first sexual intercourse
- Early age at first delivery
- High number of pregnancies
- Smoking
- Failure to be screened and treated for precancerous lesions
- Long-term use of hormonal contraceptives
- Many sexual partners; high-risk partners
- Infection with human immunodeficiency virus (HIV) or other sexually transmitted infections (e.g., herpes virus or *Chlamydia trachomatis*)
- Immunosuppression due to HIV, other diseases, chemotherapy, or other causes

Source: *National Cancer Institute www.cancer.gov/cancertopics/pdq/prevention/ cervical.*

Latest reviews indicate a close association with about 15 types of human papilloma virus (HPV infection) with cervical cancer. Types 16 and 18 are particularly linked to nearly 70% of cervical cancers. Although woman may come in contact with the virus it does not mean they will develop cancer. In fact most will shed the with little consequence. Clearly there must be other risk factors that make some women more prone to the disease. Protection against HPV infection is by using condoms during coitus. A vaccine against HPV has now been developed that is advised for adolescent girls (and boys) of 12-13 years. Although the vaccine (two approved are Gardesil-Merck and Cervarix-GSK) does not protect against all strains of HPV they appear to be effective against most of them.

Figure 18.4 illustrates the impact of HPV infection on development of cancer cervix in a developed country. A prolonged exposure is a pre-requisite for the development of cancer in vulnerable women. The incidence in this graph is plateauing after 40 years of age because if an excellent cervical screening program (Pap smear, colposcopy and treatment of pre-cancerous stage of cancer cervix).

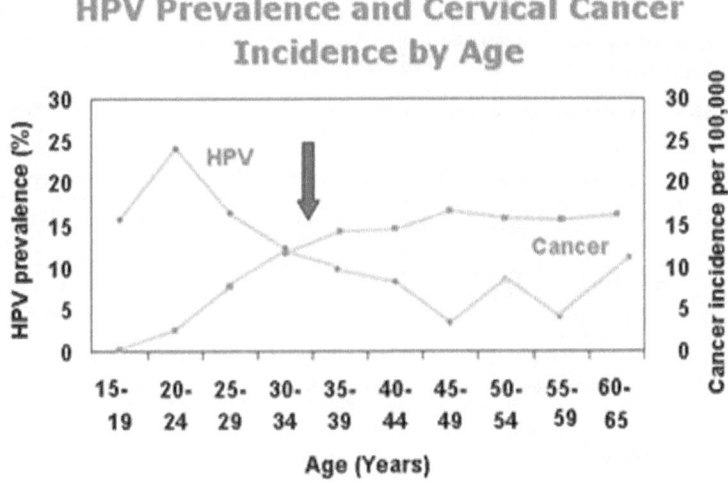

Fig. 18.3 Relationship of HPV infection and cancer of cervix

The risk factors for cancer appears to be related to women infected by not only HPV infection but also related to other sexually transmitted infections. Multiple sexual partners would increase the risk of sexually transmitted infection apart from HPV infection. These include chlamydia and herpes. Together with HPV infection, the presence of these agents almost double the risk of cancer cervix. The prolonged use of hormonal contraceptives also has been associated with an increase risk. This association is not well understood but could be related to sexual habits. The risk is doubled when the hormones have been taken for five years but after 10 years of non-use of hormone contraception, the risk almost disappears.

Chemical like benzyrene from cigarette smoke has been detected in the mucus of the cervix and could be the reason for causing cell damage in this area. Doubling of the risk of developing precancerous cells has been reported indicating a direct linkage to those who are currently smoking.

Women who have HIV AIDS have a weak immune system so do those who are on immuno-suppressive drugs like that prescribed for those who have had organ transplant. Such patients have little defense and can develop both pre-cancerous and cancerous disease of the cervix.

a.   Symptoms

There is a pre-cancerous phase in cancer of the cervix and often there is no symptom in early disease. A Pap smear can detect both pre-cancer and cancer of the cervix.

In patients with more advanced disease especially when a tumor is large enough to be seen with the naked eye, there may be bleeding between normal menstrual bleeding (intermenstrual bleeding). When the tumor is noticeably large there may be complaints of bleeding from the vagina after sexual intercourse.

Only in late stage of the disease would there be excessive bleeding from the surface of the tumor as the unhealthy tissues detach themselves from the main part of the tumor. Advanced disease is also associated with pain in the pelvis, urinary problems, ill health, loss of appetite and weight loss.

b.   Diagnosis

Early diagnosis is established by doing a pap smear. A vaginal speculum is passed into the vagina and the entire cervix is visualized. Abnormal appearance consistent with a tumor is biopsied and examined under a microscope for confirmation of cancer.

As there is a preceding pre-camcerous phase which would eventually progress to cancer, the pap smear and the colposcope have become useful diagnostic tools in detecting these early changes. Treatment of pre-cancerous disease is the most effective preventive measure in cancer of the cervix.

Treatment

Once a diagnosis is established with microscopic confirmation the patient would be counselled on the possible treatment options. After a full evaluation of the general status of the patient, she would be staged as to how far the disease has spread. Further investigations would be done to determine the extent of spread. In most instances, a CT-scan is done.

There are four stages of the disease i.e stage 1-4. For stage 1 disease, the treatment could be minimal in that only the cervix is excised under anaesthesia (CONE BIOPSY). When the disease has gone beyond that stage surgery is more extensive. Again not all patients are good candidates for surgery. Usually an extensive resection of the uterus is done with removal of the lymph nodes of the pelvis (Wertheim's hysterectomy) in Stage 1 and early stage II disease. When the disease has gone beyond a late stage of Stage 2, the patient would be given cancer drugs and radiation therapy.

What is precancerous disease of the cervix?

Cancer of the cervix is one of the few cancers that can be controlled because we know that human papilloma virus is now implicated as the cause. Moreover, this virus initiates a series of abnormal changes in the epithelial cells of the cervix that can be detected through a pap smear. These abnormal changes constitute three stages of a pre-malignant phase which can be easily determined by examining the cells from the cervix (at pap smear) and also though a magnification instrument called a colposcope. The change from pre-malignant phase to malignancy takes between 2-10 years enabling complete treatment and prevention of cancer by early detection through screening programs.

Screening the cervix through a pap smear at a gynecological examination using a vaginal speculum would permit the collection of epithelial cells from the cervical surface. These can be examined by a cytologist with the results being available after a few days. Should the results be reported as abnormal one should see a gynaecologist who then performs a colposcopy and perhaps also a biopsy where a tiny piece of tissue is taken in an outpatient clinic for further examination.

The Pap smear is by the far the most popular screening test in cancer which has been successfully employed in many developed and developing countries. In most women who do have any risk factors for cancer cervix, they are advised to have a pap smear every 3 years from 20-65 years. The intervals at which pap smear is done may vary according to the patient's life style and also the guidelines used in each country.

The pap smear is done when the woman is not menstruating. A plastic or metal speculum is passed into the vagina so that the cervix can be visualized. A wooden spatula or a plastic brush is used to take a scraping off the surface of the cervix and sent off for cytological examination.

COLPOSCOPIC EXAMINATION

Based on the results of the pap smear, a colposcopic examination may be warranted. This entails visualizing the cervix with a vaginal speculum and then directing a lighted microscope which can enlarge the area for inspection to about 20-40 times. The pattern of blood vessels and other unique changes that occur in pre-malignant and malignant state are easily recognized by an expert gynecologist. Should the area on the cervix appear suspicious of a pre-malignant disease or even look malignant a biopsy done using some local anaestheisa. This tissue is valueable for confirmation of abnormal cells and will dictate the next line of treatment after reading the report of the abnormal smear . . .

When a pap smear is reported as ABNORMAL it does not imply there is cancer. Infections and pre-malignant also are reported as abnormal. The description of the abnormal cells and if the pap smear is adequate for reporting need to be considered. The attending doctor would be able to advice as to the best form of treatment.

Most PRE-MALIGNANT disease of the cervix are treatable. Three stages of pre-malignant state are cervical intra-epithelial neoplasia, CIN 1,2,3. Most cases of CIN1 can be left alone and a repeat smear done in 6 months. CIN 2 and 3 should be surgically excised using either an electrical cautery or through surgery where a cone shaped lower part of the cervix is excised.

Frequency of pap smears

It is now generally agreed that all women (20-65years) who are sexually active should have a pap smear done regularly. In most instances a pap smear is done at three year intervals if the first two smears are normal and the woman is not at an increased risk of vaginal infections because of her life style. The attending doctor would be able to advice what intervals are best for each woman.

CANCER OF THE UTERUS

Cancer of the uterus is increasing in incidence as the life span of woman is now about 72 years in most developing countries in Asia. In 2008, slightly less than 300 000 women were diagnosed with the disease. It has become the most common gynecological cancer. Early diagnosis and treatment makes it a near curable cancer. Cancer of the endometrium (i.e the lining of the uterus, is the commonest uterine cancer. It appears to be related to unopposed action of estrogen produced in the body or consumed as hormone therapy. Progestogens usually keep the action of estrogen on the endometrial cells in check. When there is continued unopposed growth of the endometrial cells under estrogen influence, tumorous growth is seen ranging from benign polyps, excessive growth called endometrial hyperplasia or cancer of the endometrium.

A medication called TAMOXIFEN which is prescribed in breast cancer survivors is also reported to facilitate the overgrowth of endometirum (endometrial polyps, endometrial hyperplasia and endometrial cancer) when taken over a prolonged period. The obese woman, those with no children and a familial factor called LYNCH syndrome are also associated with uterine cancer.

A list of factors that are associated with cancer of the uterus is listed in Table 18.2

Table 18.1 Risk Factors for Cancer of the Uterus

Abnormal Menstruation ▪ *Irregular and infrequent menstruation (PCOS)* ▪ *Early menarche and late menopause* ▪ *Menstruating beyond 55 years of age*
Subfertile women or nulliparity
Obesity
Estrogen hormone therapy for several years with no additional progestogens
Tamoxifen treatment
Co-existing hypertension and diabetes mellitus

* PCOS-Polycystic ovary syndrome

Cancer of the endometrium develops around 60 years of age (see Fig. 18.4) as opposed to cancer of the cervix where they tend to be seen in the younger age group. This is related to the prolonged period required for the action of estrogen on the endometrium to bring on the tumor. The risk factors like unopposed estrogen action on the endometrium, irregular menstrual bleeding with infrequent cycles and obesity have all been linked to the continued exposure of unopposed estrogen acting on endometrial cells.

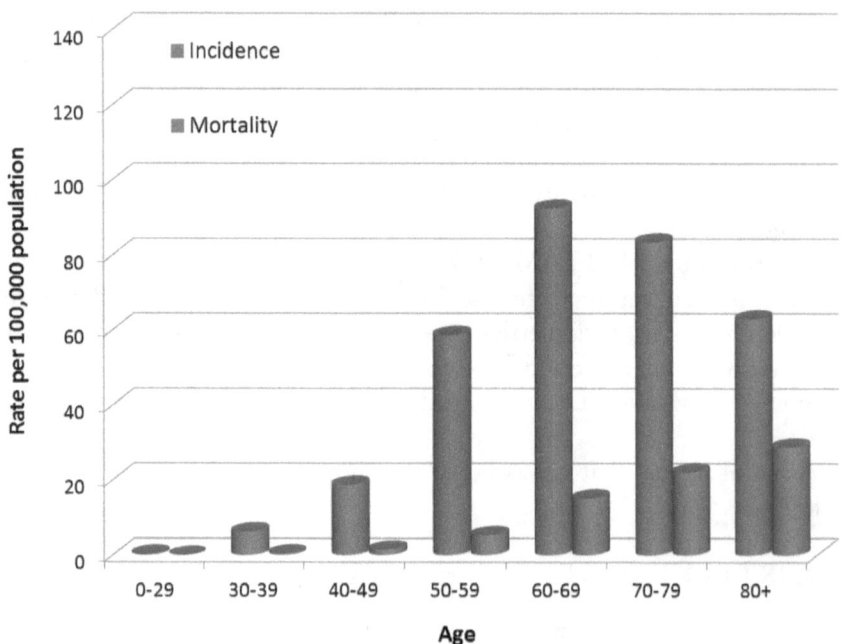

Figure 18.4 Cancer by incidence and mortality by age in the US (2007)
Source: United States Cancer Statistics (USCS): 1999-2007 Incidence and Mortality Web-based Report, released in December 2010 and available on the Centres for Disease Control and Prevention (CDC) Web site.

Symptoms

Abnormal menstrual bleeding is a common symptom in those who are around 50 years of age. As most women with cancer of the uterus are beyond the menopausal age of about 50 years, any bleeding per vaginum after attaining menopause would need a consultation and perhaps some investigations to exclude cancer of the genital tract.

In developing countries women may delay seeking a medical opinion because of modesty and ignorance. Health personnel should enquire about menstrual abnormality and also remind them of health screening according to age and risk factors. Public education and regular consultation including a pap smear would facilitate early detection of cancer.

Diagnosis

A pelvic examination would be performed in women who have abnormal bleeding around and after the menopause. Pap smears would be done, if they have not been done at regular intervals. The pap smear is not a specific test for endometrial cancer but should be part of the evaluation and is also useful for excluding abnormalities of the cervix.

Specific Investigations done for cancer of the endometrium are:

- Ultrasound of the pelvic organs
- Endometrial biopsy
- Dilatation and curettage
- Hysteroscopy

The definitive diagnosis of endometrial cancer is established by taking a specimen from the lining of the uterus (endometrium) using a small curette which can be passed through the cervical opening into the uterine cavity. This procedure can be done in the outpatient setting.

Alternatively, a hysteroscope, which is a little telescope can be passed into the uterine cavity to look for abnormal growths. If an obvious tumor is seen this is biopsied and inspected by a pathologist under the microscope. If there are no abnormal growths visualised, a scrapping of the endometrium is done to yield cells for examination in the laboratory.

In hospitals where a hysteroscope is not available, a dilatation of the cervical opening is done and the uterine cavity 'scrapped' to obtain tissues for examination.

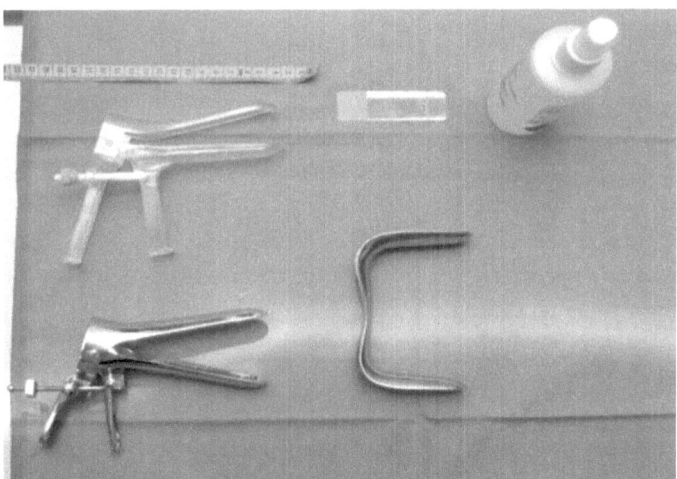

Fig.18.5 Instruments used during pelvic examination

Treatment

Once a diagnosis of cancer of the endometrium has been made the patient would need to be evaluated by a gynecologist who would determine the type of cancer she has and how far it has spread beyond the uterine cavity (staging of the tumor). Two types of cancer of the endometrium are known to occur, Type 1 which rarely spreads beyond the uterus and Type 2 which would spread quite rapidly to the lungs and other parts of the body. The latter does not have a good prognosis.

Other investigations are done to assist evaluation of the health of the patient and also to see if the tumor has spread. The CT scan of the pelvis is a common radiological examination that is done. Blood tests for assessing the full blood counts, functioning of the kidneys and liver are also done.

If the patient is anemic appropriate treatment is given. Blood transfusion may be required in some. A good meal plan should be described so that her state of nutrition would be restored to be fit for treatment.

As most patients are beyond the age of childbearing they would be counseled in having the uterus removed together with removal of the fallopian tubes and ovaries. In certain instances the lymph nodes in the pelvis would also be removed at surgery. As most patients present early (Stage 1) prognosis is good.

Other forms of treatment for cancer of the uterus

Surgical removal of the uterus, tubes and ovaries is the primary mode of treatment. Additional surgery would depend on how advanced the tumor is. Lymph nodes in the pelvis and other affected tissue may need to be removed in advanced disease.

In patient's who have disease that has spread beyond the uterus, additional treatment like radiotherapy and chemotherapy is given. Some patients may require high doses of progestogens as palliation.

Treatment of uterine cancer goes beyond surgery, chemotherapy and radiotherapy. Involving the patient in the plan of management and decision making are vital especially when the disease is advanced and overall prognosis is poor. Support from family and others together with advice on nutrition and pain relief are to be factored in.

Side-effects of treatment

a. Surgical removal of the uterus and ovaries below the age of 50 would result in menopause and perhaps symptoms related to menopause.

b. Hysterectomy is a major surgery with some risks. Hospitalization may vary from just 2 days to a few more days depending on the extent of surgery and the surgical method. Adequate counseling is essential in view of myths about surgery. Not all patients suffer from the effects of menopause. Asian women complain less about hot flashes compared to their counterparts from developed countries.

c. Sexual intercourse may be resumed once the patient has recovered from surgery and she is comfortable sexual intercourse. Coitus may be uncomfortable in women who have dry vagina due to menopause. Advice should include use of estrogen hormones or alternative therapy like vaginal lubricants and moisturizers. The desire and ability to have coitus should not be affected severely by hysterectomy.

d. Menstrual bleeding would not occur after hysterectomy.

e. Radiation treatment to the vagina and pelvis produces certain side-effects. Aim of radiation is to kill any remaining cancer cells after hysterectomy. However in the course of radiation, some of the normal cells in the vagina and neighboring organs will also be affected by the treatment resulting in a dry tight vagina (stenosis), increased frequency of urination and perhaps even bleeding at urination and passing of stools. As it is not possible to completely avoid these side effects the attending doctor would advise how these complications can be treated. Women who had radiation to the pelvis would be encouraged to have coitus to prevent the vagina becoming very narrow and tight (stenosis).

f. Skin reaction to radiation results in a mild type of 'burn'. The area of the skin exposed to radiation in the lower part of the abdomen may become red and dry. Some feel itching and burning sensation. Local soothing agents can be applied while waiting for the affected area to heal.

g. An overall feeling of fatigue and ill health often is experienced immediately after radiation and chemotherapy. Although most of these symptoms wear off over a period of time, the patient should report any symptom she experiences as all symptoms need to be evaluated by a doctor and treated accordingly.

Chemotherapy may be prescribed for women who have advanced cancer. These drugs are toxic to cancer cells but also affect normal cells. So side effects are not uncommon. These side effects depend on the type of drugs used and duration of therapy.

Loss of appetite, mouth ulcers, diarrhoea, loss of hair and decrease of circulating blood cells are well known side effects. Close monitoring of patients in specialized treatment centres is warranted.

Doctors attending cancer patients would discuss the treatment plan and what mode of treatment is appropriate. Maintaining good nutrition is vital. Emotional support and family support help victims of cancer live with cancer. Depression and anxiety should be recognized as treatable conditions and expert advice is given.

CONCLUSION

Cancer of the uterus could affect any part of the uterus. Cervical cancer and uterine (endomtrial) cancers are the common ones that affect women. Cervical cancer is seen in younger women (35-50) compared to uterine cancer which occurs largely among postmenopausal women. There is a decline in advanced cancer of the cervix in developed countries in view of effective screening like regular pap smear and health awareness programs. The introduction of HPV vaccination in adolescents is expected to see a further decline in cancer of the cervix.

Most patients with uterine cancer would complain of bleeding in the menopause. Early diagnosis of uterine cancer would get them in stage 1 of the disease which carries a good prognosis. Surgical removal of the uterus and ovaries results in good prognosis in most patients.

CHAPTER 19

CANCER OF THE OVARY—
the difficult tumor

Introduction

Cancers of the ovaries are unfortunately detected late in most instances because the disease remains silent without producing any symptoms in a majority of cases during early stage of disease. The ovaries are two little organs measuring about 1x2x3 cm lying next to the fallopian tubes close to the uterus. They are not easily reached by the examining fingers during vaginal examination unless they are large or diseased. This problem delays early detection of cancer. There are no effective screening methods for cancer of the ovary like the pap smear.

Unlike cancers of the other pelvic organs, cancers of the ovaries are a complex group of tumors because the ovary constitutes a range of specialized cells and ground substance.

Cancer of the Ovary

Cysts in the ovaries are fairly common. Most are small and are a result of follicles that grow each month under the influence of female hormones. Should ovarian cysts be small, less that 5 cm in diameter on ultrasound examination and without any features that may be suggestive of cancer, they may be left alone and re-examined after a month or so. When such cysts persist after a period of observation the doctor may suggest further tests and definitive treatment.

Because the ovaries are formed from different types of specialized cells, each type has the potential of becoming a specialized tumor. Some tumors arise from the capsule surrounding the ovaries (EPITHELIAL) while others are derived from the germ cells (TERATOMA). Both benign and malignant tumors of the ovary appear enlarged and eventually grow out of the pelvis to appear as 'mass' in the abdomen.

If the ovary is a cancer (malignant) cells from the tumor can break away from the primary site to be deposited in other parts of the body especially within the abdominal wall. Deposits of tumor may be seen in the cavity of the abdomen or involve other organs like the intestines and liver.

SYMPTOMS

Most tumors (both benign and malignant) of the ovary are found in older woman who are past 50 years. However, it may occasionally be seen in the very young and women less than 50 years. The potential for malignancy is higher when they occur in the very young and the very old.

There is limited chance of detecting an ovarian tumor if it small, by a doctor performing an physical examination of the pelvis. The chances are higher if an ultrasound is done. There is a suggestion that tumor markers for ovarian disease may be the way to go. This can be done by taking a sample of blood. However, to date this is not done as a screening measure as tumor markers may not always be present. Tumor markers are not specific for ovarian cancer i.e their appearance in blood may not indicate the presence of an ovarian cancer as it can also be positive in diseases of the ovary that are not cancerous. New research is promising in that a combination of specific tumor markers may be the way to go in screening for ovarian cancer. At the current time this sort of tumor marker screening is in the experimental stage and the tests are expensive for routine use.

Cancers of the ovaries are notorious for being silent in the early stages. No pain or vaginal bleeding are noted in most benign tumors and cancers of the ovaries. Many are detected when they have grown to a very large size in the pelvis and abdomen. Women notice that their abdominal girth has increased so as to make it difficult to wear their clothes. Some women may feel some discomfort and many more ignore these symptoms in the early stage.

Distension of the abdomen is by far the commonest complaint. Severe abdominal pain with or without fever may be noticed if the tumor has twisted on itself compromising the blood supply. In such an instance, urgent surgery is warranted.

As the tumor increases in size within the pelvis urinary disturbances may be noticed like frequent urination. This is because the tumor is pressing on the urinary bladder located in front of the uterus and ovaries. Difficulty in passing stools can be troublesome in some women.

With advancement of growth of the tumor at a later stage, there is loss of appetite and weight loss. Fluid starts accumulating in the abdomen (ASCITIS) causing further discomfort to the extent some woman find it difficult to breathe when lying flat in bed. Normal breathing movements require free excursion of the diaphragm located between the chest and abdomen. The large tumor and ASCITIS prevents easy movement of the diaphragm causing breathing difficulty.

When the tumor spreads to other parts of the body appetite is affected severely leading to weakness and lethargy. Accumulation of fluid in the chest (PLEURAL EFFUSION) would also make it very difficult to breathe easily.

It is commonly noted that very few symptoms are seen in early stage tumors of the ovary. The menstrual pattern is rarely disturbed in a majority of ovarian cancers.

Diagnosing Ovarian Tumors

The ovaries are not easily accessible for examination unlike other organs like the cervix and uterus. This makes if near impossible to directly take tissues of the tumor for sampling. An intimate examination of the pelvic organs is not a very reliable method as small tumors cannot be easily detected by the examining finger. The ultrasound may detect cysts and tumors but most women do not get regular ultrasound examination. Tumor markers have several limitations and cause unnecessary alarm as the tumor marker (from blood tests) are not specific to ovarian tumor alone. Much research is going on in detecting a combination of tumor markers in the blood but these are still early and not used for routine screening.

a.   Ultrasonogram

The ultrasound can be useful in diagnosing ovarian tumors in the pelvis and abdomen. A probe is passed into the vagina or placed on the lower part of the abdomen. High frequency sound waves produce images on a TV monitor. Echoes produced from the ultrasound transducer will hit the organs and create patterns according to its contents. In this way the pelvic organs (uterus and ovaries) are visualized. When there is fluid a different pattern is seen.

With knowledge of the disease and differing patterns of tumors, it is possible to determine if the ovary is enlarged, looks like cysts or suspicious of a tumor.

When the tumor is small a vaginal probe is used. In large tumors which have arisen into the abdomen, a larger probe placed on the abdomen (abdominal probe) is used. This abdominal probe can also be used to image the kidneys, liver and other organs in the tummy.

b. CT scan and MRI

When additional imaging is necessary a CT scan or a Magnetic Resonance Imaging (MRI) is done in the Radiology Department. These investigations require radiation (in CT scan) but produce very clear images of the whole pelvic including the muscles and all soft tissues within. They are used to visualize the tumor and the extent of involvement of other organs nearby other than the uterus and ovaries.

c. Operation required for diagnosis of ovarian cancer

The definitive method of diagnosing ovarian tumors is by surgery called a LAPAROTOMY. The patient is taken to the operating theatre and the abdomen is operated on by making a long incision over the abdomen right from the navel all the way to the bone over the pelvis. Sometimes the incision would go beyond the navel higher up the abdomen. The surgeon will have a thorough look at the tumor and extent of spread of tumor. At the same time the diseased ovaries and other organs in the pelvis like fallopian tubes and uterus are removed. In younger women who are less that 40 years, there may be a need to only remove the tumor without removing the unaffected ovary, uterus and fallopian tube. The attending doctor would have discussed these possibilities before the surgery. In selected patients minimal access surgery using laparoscopy can be done.

Staging the tumor means viewing the tumor and its extent of spread and categorizing them between Stage 1-4, four being the most advanced stage. This is done at the time of operation.

The tumor that is removed would be sent to a PATHOLOGIST who would examine the tissues under the microscope to confirm the type of tumor.

Treatment Plan

Treatment of ovarian cancer depends on the extent of spread (stage of disease), age of the patient (if she is in the postmenopausal age) and operability of the tumor.

In younger women, a more conservative approach is adopted i.e attempts are made so that only the tumor is removed at surgery if possible without removing the unaffected ovary and uterus. Such an approach would allow the woman to retain her reproductive capacity. However, should the disease be extensive so that the woman's life is at stake, the surgeon may have to remove all the internal genital organs as described above.

In older woman who have gone past the reproductive life, the usual treatment is to remove as much of the operable disease as possible. This entails removal of the ovaries and uterus together with the fallopian tubes. A 'curtain' of fat' called OMENTUM is also excised together with any other tumor bearing parts in the abdomen. The primary aim is to remove all cancerous tissue so that the final outcome is good.

Other Treatment Modalities

Surgery is the better mode of treatment. All disease should be removed at the time of surgery but this is not always possible in view of spread disease beyond the ovaries. Other modalities are required apart from surgery.

a. Chemotherapy

This modality involves the administration of anti-cancer drugs either orally or by means of injection. In most instances the medication have to be injected over a period of time through the veins through a device placed closed to a large vein in the upper chest near the heart. The drug regime would require hospitalization and close care as patient's immune system can decline rapidly during treatment. The drug is given at about 3 week intervals for about 6 cycles.

At times, the anti-cancer medication is injected directly into the tummy (INTRAPERITONEAL).

b. Radiation

Radiation treatment or radiotherapy is occasionally used a mode of treatment in ovarian cancer. Usually treatment is given for about 5 times a week for 5-6 weeks.

Intraperitoneal radiation is a form of radiation where the radioactive substance is placed close to the cancer at the time of operation thought a thin tube. This form of treatment allows the radioactive material to slowly spread throughout the abdomen and pelvis killing any cancer cells that are lurking around after removal of the tumor.

c. Biological Therapy

This is not conventional treatment but natural and artificial substances may be taken to stimulate the body's immune system to fight cancer. Such a modality is not a form of specific treatment but has been tried when all treatment modalities have failed.

SIDE-EFFECTS

Affected women are advised to seek advice from experts about specific side effects of chemotherapy and radiation treatment.

Suffice it to state that side-effects would be seen in all treatment modalities after chemotherapy and radiation treatment. These include:

a.   Problems of the Intestinal tract

- Nausea
- Vomiting
- Diarrhoea
- Mouth ulcers
- Loss of appetite

b.   Bone Marrow suppression

Blood cells in the bone marrow are markedly reduced as a result of chemotherapy and radiation. Constant monitoring of the blood cells is essential during chemotherapy.

c.   Hair loss

Hair loss is often seen after the first few cycles of chemotherapy. Patients are advised to protect the scalp by wearing hats and also wigs.

d.   Dry scaly skin

Most side effects tend to 'wear off' after completion of therapy though this may take weeks to months. As re-growth of normal cells occur there is restoration and improvement in general well being.

Follow-up and Further Care

Follow-up is essential after treatment so as to determine if the treatment given is sufficient and also to detect recurrence of tumor. Most follow-up should for prolonged periods initially at monthly intervals and later every 3-6 months.

At each visit the attending doctor will evaluate the patient and enquire about return to normal life and how eating habits have been. Weight is measured and a pelvic examination and general examination are done. Blood is also taken at periodic intervals for tumor markers and blood cell counts. The levels of tumor makers can be an indication of cure or recurrence.

CT or MRI scans may also be needed.

Menopause is another long term problem especially if the patient had both ovaries removed before natural onset of menopause. Radiation therapy and chemotherapy can also suppress the activity of functioning ovaries in the younger woman. There is a role for hormone therapy if menopausal symptoms are troublesome. This needs to be discussed with the attending doctor.

CONCLUSION

Tumors of the ovary may be benign or malignant. Most occur in the older woman and often remain silent till late stage of the tumor. Sometimes the tumor undergoes complications like twisting on itself causing abdominal pain requiring urgent surgery. There is no effective screening tool for early detection of ovarian cancer. Surgery is the primary mode of treatment for most cancers of the ovary with chemotherapy added on when surgical treatment is not optimum. Unlike other cancers of the genital tract, ovarian cancers have poorer prognosis because their first presentation with symptoms and signs often is at a late stage of cancer.

CHAPTER 20

ABNORMAL BLEEDING FROM THE UTERUS AND PRE-CANCER OF THE UTERUS

During the transition to menopause the menstrual cycles become infrequent and the flow is lighter. This is due to decline in estrogen levels which in turn is related to the follicles of the ovary becoming depleted as women move towards menopause. When the menstrual flow becomes heavier during this transition or if there is bleeding in between expected normal flow one needs to seek medical consultation. A pelvic examination is essential so as to be able to visualize the cervix and ensure it is healthy. Other abnormalities of the genital organs would need to be excluded such as an enlarged uterus, cancer of the endometrium and hormone producing tumor of the ovary (GRANULOSA CELL CANCER).

If the woman is taking hormones she should declare such history including the 'over-the-counter' prescription of 'herbal medication'. Women who are on blood thinning medication (ANTICOAGULANTS) should have the blood coagulation time determined as excessive medication can result in heavy menstrual bleeding.

Pre-cancerous conditions of the uterus

All women beyond 40 years of age who have abnormal uterine bleeding should have a thorough medical examination and all attempts are made so as to find out why such abnormal bleeding is occurring. In most instances there may not be an alarming disease to be worried about.

As has been mentioned, after menopause, although there is a rapid decline in estrogen produced by the ovaries, a weaker form of estrogen (ESTRONE) is produced as a result of conversion of androgens to estrone in the fat cells. These estrogens can stimulate the atrophic endometrium to permit abnormal growth which could become endometrial polyp, pre-cancerous endometrium or cancer.

The common types of precancerous endometrium are shown in Table 20.1.

Table 20.1 Types of Precancerous endometrium

Type of pre-cancerous growth	Risk of becoming cancer
▪ Endometrial Polyp	0
▪ Endometrial Hyperplasia	
✓ Simple without atypia	1 %
✓ Simple with atypia	8 %
✓ Complex without atypia	3 %
✓ Complex with atypia	29 %

The endometrium can also grow rather haphazardly under the influence of estrogen acting in rather 'uncontrolled manner'. (Table 20.1). These abnormal state of endometrium can arise on its own in susceptible women. It is also seen in women who have been taking tamoxifen (in breast cancer survivors) for prolonged periods and in those on estrogen hormone therapy without including 12-14 days of progestogen (combined regime).

Endometrial hyperplasia of any type or severity needs to be excluded when women bleed abnormally as they approach menopause. The disease is most commonly occurs between 50-54 years. As there is small risk of becoming cancer (see Table 20.1), early diagnosis with hysteroscopy and endometrial biopsy is a requirement.

The risk factors for endometrial hyperplasia are:

- Continuous exposure to estrogen without being opposed by progestogen
- Some uncommon familial conditions (Lynch syndrome)
- Breast cancer victims who are on tamoxifen

Diagnostic tools

a. It is again good practice to take a sample of the endometrium using a thin plastic tubing (PIPELLE curette) in women who have abnormal bleeding from the uterus as to be able to examine the tissue for the type of pre-cancerous growth or even the presence of cancer that may not be visible with a hysteroscope.

b. Other tools used are diagnostic dilatation and curettage. In this minor operation the patient would be given some anesthesia to numb the lower part of the body. The cervix is opened slightly by dilators and a metal instrument (curette) is passed through the cervical canal into the uterine cavity to obtain tissue for examination under the microscope.

c. Before these instrumentations an ultrasound examination using a vaginal probe is useful to get images of the uterus, its outline and how thick the endometrium of the uterus is. Such information helps in establishing a diagnosis and also in deciding which instrument should be used for tissue biopsy.

    The thickness of the endometrium in a postmenopausal women is rarely more than 5 mm.

d. Hysteroscopy is another method where a tiny telescope is passed into the uterine cavity to get a good view of the uterine cavity. This endoscopic image also helps in detecting the presence of polyp in the endometrium and if there are suspicious tissues that need to be biopsied. The endoscope passed into the uterine cavity could a flexible one which is about 3 mm in diameter or one that is more rigid which is 5-7 mm in diameter. The flexible endoscope is useful for outpatient viewing while the rigid endoscope requires some anaesthesia.

When performing the hysteroscopy a little fluid is pushed into the cavity first so as to distend the uterine cavity. This is necessary to facilitate viewing. As this procedure allows the surgeon to directly view the entire uterine cavity it is superior to the other tools described.

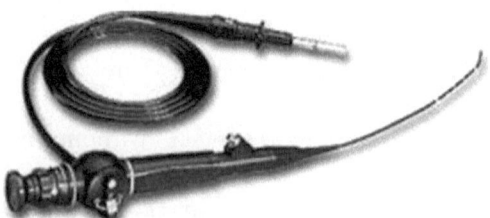

Fig. 20.1 Flexible hysteroscope
(Source: medicalexpo)

Treating Endometrial Hyperplasia

Treatment depends on the age of the patient and also the type of endometrial hyperplasia. The condition is rarely seen before 30 years of age. In the patient who has not attained menopause and the risk of cancer is low (<1%) she could be observed over for a period of time, ensuring that she has regular menstruation so that the endometrium does not growth 'unopposed". A repeat biopsy is done after six months and a decision made as to how she should be treated. If the tissue biopsy shows a worse off diagnosis and the risk of cancer is high, the patient is advised to have a hysterectomy. As most women are in the 50-54 years of age, accepting hyeterectomy as a better option is less of a problem for most women once they understand the benefits of hysterectomy.

CONCLUSION

Women past menopause should not have 'menstrual bleeding '. The transition to menopause may take several months when menstruation is lighter than normal and the cycles are in frequent. Heavy and abnormal bleeding could be due to several other causes. Endometrial hyperplasia and endometrial polyps are two of such. Endometrial hyperplasia is a pre-cancerous condition that requires treatment. In the severe form there is high risk for development of endometrial cancer. As most women are between 50-54 years, hysterectomy may be the better option.

Doctor, I have a problem . . . .

I am 52 years and have been having regular pap smears after menopause. The last smear showed some abnormal endometrial cells.

What should I do?

Answer: It is not unusual to get endometrial cells on pap smear though the pap smear was designed as a screening tool for cervical cancer.

Do you have any bleeding after menopause?.

In any case you would require a thorough examination which may include performing a repeat pap smear, colposcopy and also hysteroscopy and biopsy of the inner lining of the cervical canal and uterine cavity (endometrium).

CHAPTER 21

THE DRY VAGINA

Postmenopause is categorized as early in the first 1-4 years and late after that. In the early phase hot flashes are more prominent. However, with further depletion of estrogen due to atrophy of the ovaries changes in other organs in the pelvis become evident. One of it is the 'dry vagina' or better referred as 'ATROPHIC VAGINITIS or POSTMENOPAUSAL VAGINITIS.

Estrogen is vital to keep the mucosa of the vagina moist and healthy sustaining the pH at an acidic medium. There are tiny particles in the cells of the vagina called 'receptors' which assist in engaging the estrogens to the cells surface to maintain the healthy eco-system within the vagina. The mucosa becomes thin and non-elastic with depletion of estrogen resulting in a variety of local changes. The pH and the 'good' bacteria within the vagina are replaced with a higher pH and potential for pathogens to invade the vaginal mucosa. The loss of elasticity will cause the vagina to become tighter. Together with a loss of moistness, sexual intercourse becomes difficult and even painful.

The narrow and shortened vagina is often the reason why postmenopausal women refrain from sexual practices. The thinned surface can be easily traumatized even by cleaning or at intercourse resulting in vaginal bleeding. As time goes on sexual intercourse is almost impossible.

SYMPTOMS

Itching of the vagina associated with a stinging burning sensation is commonly complained of. Vaginal dryness is a prominent feature. Burning sensation may be felt after urination when some of the acid urine trickles onto the vaginal surface.

Progressive loss of both collagen and elastin, the supportive tissues of the vagina are both lost markedly in the postmenopause period. The lubricating fluid within the vagina is lost eventually, the cause for vaginal dryness. The tiny blood vessels underlying the mucous of the vagina also atrophy giving the vagina a rather 'parchment paper' pale look. The underlying support tissues of the vulva is also lost leading to a thin and atrophic vulva.

The skin overlying the vulva appears rough and flaccid and pubic hair becomes sparse. The lining of the bladder wall is also affected by depletion of estrogen. This explains the reason for a reduction in the volume of the bladder and its inability to store a larger volume of urine as they did in younger life. Urinary symptoms like increase in the frequency of urination and loss of urine at coughing are not uncommon in the older woman.

In the fertile period of life, estrogen is plentiful and the vagina is well lubricated in the presence of friendly bacteria called 'Doderlein lactobacilli'. This bacteria provides the acid medium for the vagina and also protects the vagina from invasion by pathogens. A change of environment occurs after estrogen depletion making it prone for bacteria from surrounding organs especially from the skin of the perineum, anus and rectum, to find its way into the vagina. One of the hygienic means of cleaning the perineum and vulva is to clean from the front to the back. Doing it the other way round is one of the reasons bacteria from the anus and rectum find their way to the vagina. Bacteria can also come from the bladder and urethra in front of the vagina. Should these pathogens eventually find their way in the vagina, an infection would occur leading to vaginal discharge, itchiness and burning sensation.

Bacteria can also find its way up the urinary tract causing infection of the bladder resulting in burning sensation at urination and also increased frequency of urination.

The vulnerability of the vagina at menopause and the rapid change in the 'ecosystem' of the vagina permit the growth of fungal infections called 'THRUSH OF CANDIDIASIS'. This is a common fungal infection seen in about 50% of women beyond 60 years. These are more prevalent in those who also suffer from poorly controlled diabetes mellitus.

TREATMENT

All women who have vaginal discomfort should have a pelvic examination done. Care is taken when a vaginal speculum is passed into the vagina as the vagina is both dry and narrow making it not possible to use the normal vaginal speculums. The vagina is not only dry and narrow but it is also shorter in length in postmenopausal women as it retracts in size.

Pap smears are usually taken from the cervix if this has not been done before. The vagina is inspected for the presence of infections and any other disease especially if the patient complained of postmenopausal bleeding.

Atrophic vaginitis is best treated with estrogen creams applied locally or by using an estrogen ring inserted into the vagina. The attending doctor would advice as to the best mode of application. Current thoughts are that local application of estrogen is preferred. Other modes of application is by applying the estrogen on the skin. Unless indicated, rarely is oral estrogen prescribed for atrophic vaginitis.

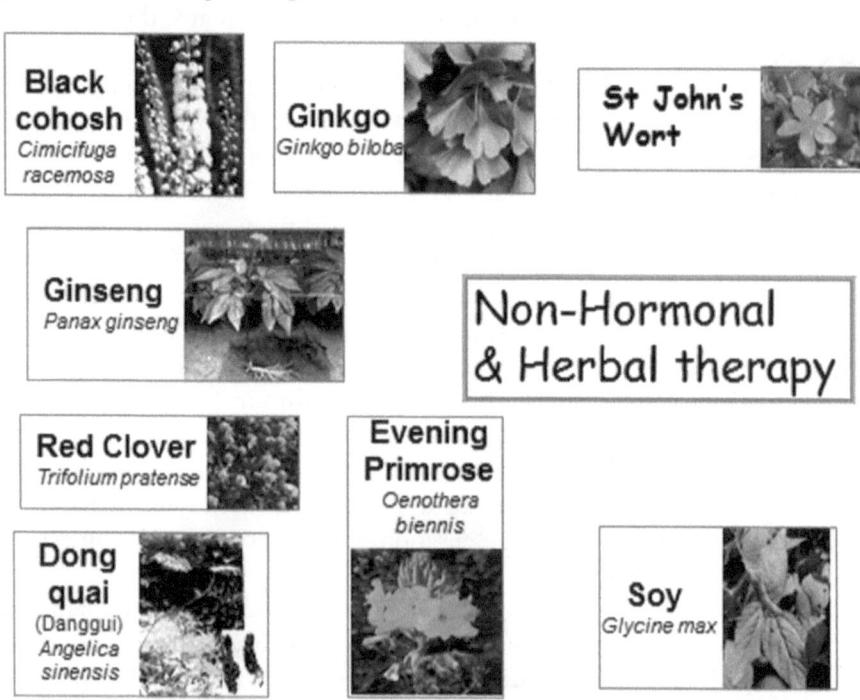

Fig.21.2: Alternative Therapy and Bioidentical Medication

Table 21.1 Estrogen applications

Vaginal cream
■ soothing   ■ can be messy
Silastic vaginal rings

■ convenient as it is placed 3 monthly
   ■ sensed during intercourse
   ■ may be expelled during defecation of urination
   ■ some have vaginal discharge

Vaginal tablets (inserted into vagina)
■ less messy than cream   ■ placed twice weekly (so may forget)

A little cotton bud mounted on a wooden stick is used to take swabs from the wall of the vagina. This is sent to the laboratory to look for offending bacteria that is causing the problem. Experienced doctors can make a diagnosis of THRUSH by looking at the nature of the vagina if this fungus is present in large amount. Treatment for thrush is quite simple. Either pessaries of the medication or tablets may be prescribed. These are inserted into the vagina

Urinary symptoms would require examination of the urine. The bacteria causing the infection will be evident within 3 days of culturing the urine. Urinary antispetics are given according to the type of bacteria that is seen on urine culture.

PSYCHOSEXUAL PROBLEMS

Painful and difficult sexual intercourse due to atrophic vaginitis can be a cause for concern as it affects both the life of the woman and her spouse. As the vaginal is atrophic and dry treatment is available by way if estrogen and lubricants.

A frank discussion is warranted about the likes and dislikes of sexual health and if atrophic vagina and pain at sexual intercourse are the reasons for refraining from coitus. Current lifestyle favours a healthy relationship in a couple including sexual health. The couple are explained on the treatment modalities and how such can be used. If the patient is not happy with estrogens she could be advised on the value of lubricants that would enable a reasonable sexual union with little discomfort. It is a well known fact that regular coitus would also prevent the vagina from further narrowing and retracting to become smaller in length.

Psychosexual health is integral to happy relationships and this dimension should be explored. If the spouse is physically impaired as a result of ailments like stroke, one should consult a psychologist or sex therapist who could advice more about sexual happiness.

Both painful intercourse and urinary problems contributes to loss of self esteem and withdrawal from society. There are remediable measures that would improve quality of life and such treatment should not be denied because the woman is past the menopause. Estrogen therapy used as skin applications and by applying to the vagina appears to be safe options and are well accepted by many women. It restores moistness of the vagina enabling comfortable sexual intercourse. Resumption of coitus has positive impact on women. preventing the psychosexual health

Lubricants, when used should be water soluble and not oil based. The lubricant can be applied both the penis and also into the vagina before coitus. Lubricants like liquid paraffin and vegetable oil should not be used. Preparatory lubricants like K-Y jelly (Johnson-Johnson) is innocuous and odourless and does not stain clothes.

Table 21.2 Suggested steps in treating atrophic vaginitis

- Re-look at your lifestyle and see it there is a need to modify it should it not be suitable for healthy living in this age (reduce weight, select your food carefully)
- Discussion with spouse on intimate relationships and shortcomings
- Stop smoking as it worsens vaginal atrophy
- Consult your physician for vaginal atrophy (use of estrogen and/or water soluble lubricant
- Sexual health may be important to you and your spouse, address this with experts
- Quality of life issues need to be addressed, so put in place strategies to overcome stressors, depression, sexual health, relationship problems and individual needs
- Treat chronic diseases and conditions that are related to the postmenopuasal age (urinary incontinence, urinary infection)

Conclusion

Atrophic vaginitis is a direct effect of estrogen decline at menopause. It can cause dry vagina, itchiness and painful intercourse. If vaginal bleeding occurs the woman should be thoroughly examined. In other instances treatment by way of estrogen creams and water soluble lubricants are useful in improving quality of life. Estrogen creams are superior in restoring the moistness of the vagina. Regular coitus prevents narrowing of the vagina.

CHAPTER 22

PROLAPSE OF THE UTERUS AND URINE INCONTINENCE

Apart from playing an integral role in maintaining feminity, estrogen has a vital role in maintaining collagen and elastin in many parts of the body. The uterus, vagina, urinary bladder and rectum in the pelvis are supported by a network of muscles and thick string like tissues called ligaments which contain proteineous materials called collagen and elastin. After menopause the quality of collagen and elastin is affected. Loss of quality of the supporting ligaments together with weakness of the supporting muscles, prolapse of the genital organs and other pelvic organs are apparent in some women.

When one or more of these organs slip down from its normal location into the vagina because of weakness of the support PELVIC ORGAN PROLAPSE occurs. Other words used are UTERO-VAGINAL PROLAPSE and PROCIDENTIA.

Another common problem complained of is the involuntary leakage of urine in older woman. Both pelvic organ prolapse POP and urine leakage may be seen occurring together in some women

PROLAPSE OF THE UTERUS AND VAGINA

The female genital organs consist of the vulva and vagina externally and uterus, fallopina tubes and ovaries lying internally within the pelvis suspended by ligaments attached to the bones in the pelvis. These organs at tucked between the urinary bladder and urethra infront and rectum and anus behind.

The greater part of the uterus is lying within the pelvis supported by a tough muscle called the PELVIC FLOOR MUSCLE with added support provided by ligaments and fascia. The urinary bladder and rectum are also supported by this muscle, ligaments and fascia. The supporting tissues withstand various types of insult through the years of standing upright and from the straining involved in childbirth. Among women who suffer some degree of POP, 50 % have had vaginal childbirth. Chronic cough and obesity can also stress the supporting muscles, ligaments and facsia. Another two factors that can negatively impact on the supporting pelvic floor muscle and ligaments are loss of strength of the supports due to ageing and much more important is the rapid decline in estrogen which has a positive influence on collagen. POP also is seen after hysterectomy.

Fortunately, not all women complain of POP as they go past menopause. It looks like some women are more susceptible than others despite all the factors mentioned including the childbirth and obesity. Perhaps some women are already predisposed to POP.

Types of Prolapse of Genital Organ in Women

Various grades of genital prolapse are known. All depends on the extent of 'slipping' through into and past the vagina. In 'procidentia' the entire uterus descends through and out of the vagina presenting as 'mass' outside the vulva. This mass can be easily replaced within the vagina but tends to 'fall' out again when she strains at passing urine or at defecation.

The types of POP and common symptoms women complain of are is shown in Table 22.1 Symptoms may vary depending on the severity of prolapse and the organs involved.

Table 22.1 Pelvic organ prolapse and common symptoms

Common Symptoms	Type of Pelvic Organ Prolapse
▪ A vague sensation of 'something coming down' through the vagina ▪ A feeling of fullness within the vagina ▪ Difficulty during sexual intercourse or unable to have (due to procidentia) ▪ Associated with urine leakage when coughing, sneezing or brisk exercise	▪ Utero-vaginal prolapse— uterus passing out of vagina ▪ Cystocele—part of the bladder is pushed through the vagina ▪ Enterocele—part of intestine is pushed through vagina ▪ Rectocele-part of the rectum is pushed

In the early stage of prolapse the uterus slips out of the supports but stays within the vagina. Women tend to complain of 'something coming down' and the diagnosis is clinched when a pelvic examination is done. With time this degree of prolapse could become more severe so as to be obvious when the woman strains to defecate. In procidentia the prolapsed uterus 'drops' out of the vagina completely and needs to be gently pushed back into the vagina with fingers. In neglected cases ulcers can develop in the dependent part of the prolapsed uterus outside. Rarely the tissues surrounding become swollen causing the prolapse to become incarcerated.

Table 22.2 Stages of Genital Organ Prolapse

Stage of Prolapse	
1	Prolapse is more than 1cm above the opening of the vagina
2	Prolapse is 1cm or less from the opening of the vagina
3	Prolapse sticks out of the vagina opening more than 1cm, but not fully
4	The full length of the prolapse bulges out of the vagina

Associated Problems

As the uterus is closely associated with other organs nearby when prolapse of the uterus occurs it is not unusual to see the other organs prolapse with it. These are shown in Table 22.2. The main issue is weakness of the support and it is obvious that the urinary bladder in front and the rectum behind push down the vagina givng rise to various terms included in the table. Symptoms specific to the prolapse of the urinary bladder are increased frequency of urination and in severe cases there is difficulty in emptying the bladder. Constipation and difficulty in emptying the rectum are seen when there is a RECTOCELE. Women have been known to use their fingers placed within the vagina to evacuate the constipated stools.

a. Vagina

The vagina is a muscular organ between the vulva and uterus. The cervix, the neck of the uterus projects into the vagina. In early stage of uterine prolapse the cervix tends to be a little longer and with further laxity of the supports will go past the opening of the vagina together with the uterus.

b. Urinary bladder

Since the urinary bladder is just in front of the vagina and uterus, a portion of the bladder which is in close contact will descend as the uterus descends. This is noticed during a pelvic examination. Such a prolapse where the predominant bulge is the urinary bladder is called a CYSTOCELE.

c. Rectum

In a similar fashion, the gut and rectum that are in close proximity to the back of the vagina can also bulge into the vagina. This type of prolapse can occur together with uterine prolapse or by itself. When the gut prolapses through, the term ENTEROCELE is used while RECTOCELE is present with prolapse of the rectum.

SYMPTOMS

Prolapse of the genital tract is not peculiar to menopause alone. It has occasionally seen in younger women in the childbearing years. A congenital weakness of the support of the uterus is probably the reason younger women have genital organ prolapse.

However, far more women with genital organ prolapse are in the postmenopausal age. Most women would complain of 'something coming down the vagina' in the beginning. This discomfort varies according to the severity of prolapse. When the uterus or adjoining organs prolapse out of the vagina, the diagnosis is apparent.

Associated symptoms are related to the presence of enterocele and rectocele.

Sexual Intercourse

There are several reasons why sexual intercourse may not be as frequent as before menopause. The discussion in Chapter 21 on atrophic vagina relates to dry vagina making intercourse painful. In pelvic organ prolapse sexual intercourse is possible in early stages of the problem. But when the prolapse is of higher degree especially in procidentia, sexual intercourse becomes awkward and difficult. In advanced degrees pf prolapse the woman may refrain from coitus altogether.

Treatment of pelvic organ prolapse enables resumption of sexual intercourse provided atrophic vagina is also treated appropriately.

TREATMENT of Prolapse of the Genital Organs

As genital organ prolapse is a form of hernia it is possible to treat the condition both surgically or by insertion of devices to hold the uterus within the vagina. Several health issues need to be dealt with before definitve treatment is given. As age related disease are seen in the postmenopausal years, it is vital to attend to treating such disease ailments before contemplating surgery.

Factors that will need to be considered in dealing with treatment of POP are:

- Age
- Menopausal symptoms
- Pre-existing medical and surgical disease
- Medication the patient is on for such diseases
- Weight and exercise programs she is familiar with

a. Age

Age is not a barrier to surgical treatment of POP. Quality of life is restored with surgery. Surgical repair of POP is done when the woman is surgically fit i.e all pre-existing disease are well controlled. In the younger woman there is a need to save the uterus and hence repair of the defects and restoration of the supports only is done. In the postmenopausal woman, the uterus is small because of atrophy and the ovaries are also not functioning The most appropriate surgical treatment would then be removal of the uterus and ovaries through the vagina and repair of the defects of the pelvic floor tissues.

b. Menopausal symptoms

When treating POP symptoms of menopause should also be treated. If the patient has menopasual symptoms like hot flashes and urinary symptoms these should be addressed. Urinary infections are treated completely before performing surgery for POP. If the patient has leakage of urine which requires a surgical approach this needs to be discussed with her prior to surgery for POP as both surgeries can be done at the same sitting. Correction of urinary incontinence due to coughing and sneezing requires additional support surgery after completion of the operation for POP (i.e COLPOSUSPENSION).

Hormone therapy may be warranted in women who do not have any contraindications to its use. Local application of estrogen restores turgidity of the mucosa of the vaginal wall.

c. Pre-existing disease

Certain disorders like a chronic cough due to smoking and obesity strain the pelvic floor muscles and supports of the genital organs. This is not good for a woman with POP. She should be advised to cease smoking and seek help in improving her lung functions. Weight loss regimes are beneficial in the long run and should be encouraged. Attempts at losing weight prior to surgery for POP would prevent recurrence of POP.

POP is a nuisance rather than being a fatal disease. Seldom do women die as a result of POP. This is the reason for planning surgery for POP after ensuring the patient's pre-existing disease like diabetes mellitus and hypertension are well controlled and that she is fit for surgery. The opinion of the physician is required for adequate management of medical disease. If the patient has a risk for developing a stroke or a coronary heart disease, she should be evaluated and appropriate counseling given together with advice when surgery for POP is to be done. There is no urgency for surgery.

In the meantime the POP could be managed by inserting a ring pessary which would keep the prolapse reduced temporarily.

d. Treatment options for pelvic organ prolapse

POP is largely treated by surgery just as one does surgery for a hernia. However, as mentioned above, in woman who are not fit for surgery or do not want it, one could offer a ring pessary.

Non-surgical Treatment

If the vagina is dry local application of estrogen cream for about two weeks is advised prior to surgery.

If there is an ulcer on the edge of the prolapse uterus (DECUBITUS ULCER) the prolapse is reduced and held within the vagina with a ring pessary and the ulcer treated with local medication. If there is infection appropriate antibiotics are prescribed. The patient is taught how to remove the ring pessary and re-insert it. The ring pessary is removed and cleaned before re-insertion. The vagina is inspected for any pressure sores that may have developed because of the ring pessary.

Ring pessaries are also useful (as mentioned) in women who are not keen of surgery or a awaiting palnned surgery. The ring pessary is a soft elastic silastic device which is inserted into the vagina after having pushed back the prolapsed organ into the vagina. The ring unfolds itself within the vagina abutting against the upper wall of the vagina so as to keep the prolapse uterus within.

A woman using ring pessaries are advised to check if the ring is expelled when she strains at urination of defecates. Should it fall out it should be cleaned before re-insertion.

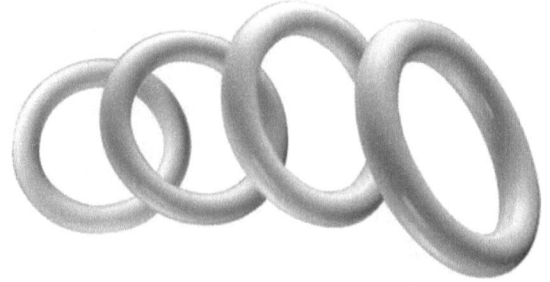

Fig. 22.1 Silastic Ring Pessary
Source: www.smith-medical com.

Surgical Treatment

As far as surgical treatment goes, women will be offered two surgical procedures:

- Vaginal hysterectomy with repair of the pelvic floor
- Manchester repair

The Manchester repair is not commonly done nowadays. It is a useful procedure in the younger woman who needs to retain the uterus. This operation entails surgical removal of the elongated cervix and tightening procedure to enhance the supports of the uterus. Redundant tissues around the vagina is excised and any defect in the supports is reinforced. If there is a cystocele or rectocele, these are also repaired at the same sitting.

In vaginal hysterectomy the supports of the uterus are excised through the vagina and the uterus removed. The remaining supports are reinforced and strengthened as the upper vaginal opening created at the beginning of surgery is closed to prevent any contents of the pelvis from herniating. Again if the patient has an associated cystocele, enterocele or rectocele, these are repaired in turn.

If the patient has urinary incontinence (STRESS URINARY INCONTINENCE) she would require additional support surgery. Current treatment is to insert a tape so as to support the neck of the urinary bladder leading to cure if urine incontinence on coughing or sneezing.

After the surgery for POP a urinary catheter would be left for a day or so. The vagina is packed with a roller gauze immediately after completion of the operation.

Patients who have had surgery for POP tend to be hospitalized for a few days before they are discharged. In most instances regional anesthesia (injection over the low back so as numb the lower part of the body) is sufficient to complete the operation. A small catheter to administer the anesthetic drug in the spine (EPIDURAL) is also useful to give pain relief after the surgery while the patient is recovering in the hospital. Most patients would not need epidural anesthesia for more than a day. The roller gauze placed in the vagina is removed the next day and so is the urinary catheter.

Surgery through the vagina is well tolerated by patients as pain is not as much as if one would have with surgery through the abdomen. Recovery is also much faster. The wound within the vagina also heals much faster. Most women would be reviewed by the doctor after 4-6 weeks. She is advised to resume her normal activities including sexual intercourse (if she desires) in about 3 months.

After surgery women are advised not to carry heavy weights lest they strain the pelvic floor. Constipation would also cause strain to the pelvic floor and stool softeners and high roughage food are advised. All activities that places undue strain on the pelvic floor is discouraged. She may be advised to resume hormone therapy if it is indicated.

Other types of surgery

i.   Laparoscopic surgery
ii. Vaginal vault surgery

In some patients prolapse of the uterus is done through a laparoscope where the uterus (or prolapsed vaginal vault) is strung up against the lower part of the backbone within the abdominal cavity suing an artificial tape. Vaginal vault prolapse occurs in some women who have had hysterectomy for a gynecological problem earlier. This prolapse can be operated on vaginally by stitching the high end of the vault wihin the ligaments of the pelvis. Alternatively the vault can be suspended to the backbone as described.

e. Exercise

Exercise is central to life in postmenopausal age. Regular exercise maintains weight and improves functioning of the heart. Exercise can all be directed to strengthen the pelvic floor muscles and has been shown to improve symptoms due to both POP and urine loss at sneezing and coughing.

Specific exercise to the pelvic floor is called Kegel's exercise. A device called Kegel's perineometer has a pressure gauge attached to it. The long arm of the instrument is inserted into the vagina as the muscles in the vagina are voluntarily squeezed, the pressure gauge will indicate the success of the exercise. This motivates the woman to continue to focus on strengthening the pelvic muscles. The exercise is done for about 10-15 minutes about 2-3 times a day. This method is said to indicate success of the exercise in an objective way.

An alternative to this is the insertion of vaginal cones (Fig. 22.3). The aim is to perform the exercises as attempts are made to retain the cones within the vagina.

Although there are merits to the use of the instrument, many conservative women are not comfortable in placing the instrument into the vagina as described.

A similar less objective means of pelvic floor exercise is to teach women how the exercise is done using pictorial diagrams. Such exercise is commonly performed in postnatal classes. Pelvic floor exercise is beneficial for all women and should be taught as part of wellness.

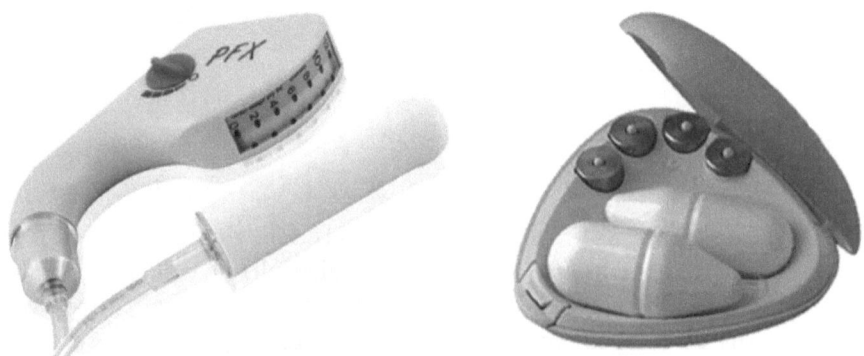

Fig. 22.2 Kegel Perineometer and Vaginal Cones
Source: www. Win-health.com

LEAKING URINE

The primary function of the urinary bladder is to store urine and empty it at appropriate intervals when the desire to urinate occurs. With the onset of menopause the bladder undergoes some adaptations which result in a smaller capacity so that there is need to empty the bladder more frequently. However, when one has to go to the toilet more often than about eight times a day or if sleep is disturbed because of the need to empty the bladder one needs to investigate for urine infection which is a problem in the menopause.

Involuntary urine leakage can also occur as a result of some surgical complication after hysterectomy or following cancer of the cervix. In these instances there is a communication that is artificailly created between the bladder and the vagina which result in continuous flow of urine. It is called a FISTULA and would not be discussed in detail in this section.

Two other conditions that are peculiarly seen around the menopausal age where urine leaks without being able to control voluntarily are:

a.   Urge incontinence
b.   Genuine stress incontinence

The urinary bladder is a very versatile organ working under the influence of the nervous system. It is able to store up to 150 ml of urine without a woman sensing it is there but beyond that she is able to tolerate accumulating amounts up to 450 to 500ml. This capacity is less in the postmenopausal period. When the maximum capacity is reached there is a sensation to pass urine. Under normal circumstances one can delay passing urine till we find a suitable place and time to urinate. The bladder muscle can be controlled to some extent. This degree of independence is exerted by nerve stimulations of the bladder muscle from the spinal cord and brain.

a.   Urge Incontinence (overactive bladder)

As mentioned above the bladder capacity is smaller in the menopausal years with some degree of thinning of the bladder wall as estrogen declines. The smaller bladder capacity is also associated with a more sensitive bladder muscle (DETRUSOR MUSCLES). If there is a bladder infection local sensitivity of bladder muscle is increased tremendously so as increase the urge to empty the bladder. The woman tends to urinate more frequently and sleep may also be disturbed. In some women the sensitivity of the bladder is so high that she has the urge to empty the bladder even if there is no bladder infections. The urgency is so great that she will not be able to make it to the toilet leaking urine and wetting her underclothes in the process. The involuntary loss of urine in this instance is called URGE INCONTINENCE or 'overactive bladder'. It is said the main problem is due to the oversensitivity of bladder muscles (DETRUSOR OVERACTIVITY). The cause of urge incontinence is not known but remains a nuisance as the bladder contract even when the bladder is not full and urine is passed with the woman having no control.

Table 22.3 Signs of Urge Incontinence

- Urgency : sudden desire to pass urine without being able to put off or delay
- Frequency: going to the toilet more than 8 times a day
- Nocturia: having to wake up at night to pass urine
- Urge incontinence: leakage of urine before making it to the toilet

In order to diagnose 'urge incontinence' a written record of daily urine passing habits is asked for including the consumption of water for the day and what beverages are taken. This is called a BLADDER DIARY. The record for three days is required. The urine is checked for infection as bladder infection is a common cause of such urgency of passing urine. In a urine infections is present appropriate antibiotics are given and the woman is seen for persistence of urge incontinence. Should the symptoms persist than further investigations are done.

One of the ways to confirm if the bladder muscles are very sensitive (typical of urge incontinence) is to measure the pressure of the bladder by inserting small electrodes into the bladder through the urethra. This is connected to a measuring instrument as a graph is produced as water fills up the bladder slowly. This whole test is called a FILLING CYSTOMETRY. Oversensitive detrusor muscles show typical abnormal wave pattern on a graph that is generated by the machine.

TREATMENT of URGE INCONTINENCE

Some beverages like coffee and tea are known to worsen urge incontinence. It is advised that these be limited as much as possible. Cola and alcohol are also known to 'irritate' the bladder. Hence, it also advisable to make changes to our lifestyles to try to omit these drinks. All forms of caffeine have a diuretic effect apart from stimulating the bladder muscles.

Limiting water consumption at night, say after dinner at 8 pm would reduce the functioning of the kidneys and less urine would trickle into the bladder at night so not to have to get up at night to pass urine. One should also try to reduce the total water intake to about 6-8 cups or less than 2 litres a day if possible.

Bladder training is a good measure that can be learnt through practice. Some women have the wrong notion that by going to the toilet more often they can overcome the problem. The bladder needs to be trained to hold a larger volume of urine. This can be achieved by delaying the need each time through mental distraction for periods of 10 minutes or more. With more practice, the duration of delay can be increased slowly to 15 min and half an hour.

Pelvic floor exercises has been shown to improve symptoms due to urge incontinence.

Medications could improve symptoms., These directly act on detrusor muscles of the bladder suppressing its action to variable extents. Side effects may be troublesome and consultation is required. As drug interaction can be an issues as many women may be on other medications for age related diseases this should be discussed with the doctor.

BLADDER TRAINING (DRILL)

The bladder is taught to slowly stretch so as to hold larger volumes of urine.

- Aim is to establish more control over bladder activity by slowly increasing the timing of urine passing and delaying desire to pass urine
- Maintain a diary so as to establish a baseline for the first three days

  o Note uncontrolled urine leakage, fluid consumed and bladder irritants (caffeine, alcohol, diuretics)
  o Also measure urine passed by keeping a measuring jar (incontinence nurse should be able assist)

- Consider that increasing the durations of passing urine are achievements.

  o Log in for the first three days as usual to get an idea of normal habits
  o Later discover how often you go to toilet (hourly etc) and how much you pass (150ml) each time
  o Then learn to hold urine longer than interval recorded before
  o Learn to distract yourself to improve on 'delay time'

    - Sitting up and crossing the legs

- Perform pelvic floor exercise
- Think of unrelated matters like a movie or do SUDOKU

Bladder training requires commitment as it is tedious and requires patience. The training should go on for weeks to months as the detrusor muscles do not respond so quickly. It needs support of the continence nurse or doctor so that the woman would persevere with the training to get best results. Bladder training should be done even if she is taking medication for urge incontinence. Some patients may not need medication as bladder training may produce a reasonable quality of life.

Medication for urge incontinence

When bladder training is ineffective or does not give reasonable improvement medications called 'anticholinergics' are prescribed. Commonly used medications are:

- Oxybutinin
- Tolterodine
- Trospimum chloride
- Propiverine
- Soliferacin

All of them are known to relax the bladder muscle. Side effects are less with the newer generation of medication. One is advised to take the medication for about six months initially and if good improvement is noticed, may stop it to see if the problem is still present. Together with bladder training most women improve reasonably. Should symptoms return medication is resumed.

Common side effects are dry mouth, blurred vision and constipation.

Other forms of Treatment

Other forms of treatment are not commonly resorted to. Very rarely does one need some form of augmentation surgery of the urinary bladder to increase the size so as to hold a larger volume of urine. Even if such an operation is done there will be difficulty in emptying the bladder and one need to learn how to catheterize herself.

Nerve stimulation using a small electrical device implanted under the skin over the buttocks so as effect the sacral nerve has been used to control the bladder with varying success. Injection of botulinum toxin A into the bladder muscles is a new method that require more evaluation before recommending them for routine use.

When everything mentioned fails the ureters (that is the tube that facilitates trickling g of urine from kidney into the bladder) is re-routed into a short segment of the intestine and then connected to the skin surface. This procedure call URINARY DIVERSION is rarely required.

b. Genuine Stress Incontinence

Urine seldom leaks out during period of coughing and sneezing as the bladder is well supported above the pelvic floor muscles and is designed to keep the bladder sphincters closed during such strenuous periods. The neck of the urinary bladder is invested with good muscle fibers which would keep it closed tightly when there is a cough. It is not unusual to have a spurt of urine escaping intentionally when the bladder is full and there is a sudden cough. However, the infrequent occurrence of such instances is not to be concerned about.

Genuine stress incontinence is a form of urine loss that occurs only with some strenuous activity. This is often due to weakening of the pelvic floor support. Vaginal childbirth appears to be associated with this problem. In genuine stress incontinence the woman tends to lose spurts of urine each time she coughs sneezes or does some strenuous work wetting her under clothes. She has not control over this. She is unable to retain urine even if she wants to. This can be both embarrassing and uncomfortable so much as to affect her normal routines.

Symptoms

The main symptoms are the sudden loss of urine coming in spurts each time she exercises, coughs or sneezes. This is quite different from urge incontinence as the bladder muscles work well and are not overactive. It is thought that about 15 % of women beyond 40 years would have some degree of stress incontinence making it a fairly common problem in the post-menopausal age.

In a third of women both stress incontinence and urge incontinence occurs.

Diagnosis

The diagnosis is strongly made with direct observation of the urine spurting at a pelvic examination. Sometimes it is not possible to observe the event. Other tests are done. One simple test is to ask the woman to wear a pre-weighed sanitary pad and instruct her to go up and down a staircase for a while and inspect the pads for wetting. Another way is to place her over a piece of paper and ask her to cough repeatedly or jump up and down and look for wetting the paper beneath her.

A more sophisticated method is to do urodynamic tests in a clinic setting as was described under FILLING CYSTOMETRY. In this instance, as one is measuring the pressure of the urinary bladder, the patient is also asked to cough as the bladder is being filled with water. Leaking of urine is looked for with each cough.

TREATMENT

Pelvic floor muscle exercise and surgery to support the bladder outlet are the main modes of treatment. Other forms of treatment are not commonly done as success rates to become continent are high with these two measures.

a.   Pelvic floor exercise

Nearly 50% of women report good results after about 6 months of pelvic floor exercise. The exercise is best supervised by a physiotherapist in the beginning before the patient does it on her own. This is because the correct muscles need to be strengthened. Weight reduction if the women are over-weight improves the outcome of exercise. The basic steps of pelvic floor exercise is outlined in the table below.

Pelvic floor exercise

- Sit on chair comfortably with feet resting on ground and knees apart
- Squeeze pelvic muscles (the focus is on the pelvic muscle, as if one is stopping urine or flatus from passing midway)
- Notice action of appropriate pelvic muscle
- Exercises are repeatedly done without moving either the buttocks or legs
- Although the use of vaginal cones or Kegel device helps one to be more focussed in the pelvic muscle to be strengthened women who are not comfortable with these devices may elect to do the exercise without them
- The physiotherapist who is instructing you may offer alternatives for focussing on pelvic muscle strengthening like inserting a finger into the vagina to feel the squeeze of the muscle onto the finger within the vagina
- Each 'squeeze' is held for about 5-10 seconds, repeating the process after relaxing for about five times. The ultimate aim is experience two specific phases in the exercise, a pull up phase and a period of relaxation. This is vital for positive results.
- The whole process is then repeated more quickly (for another five times) so as to experience the rapid pull ups (first phase). (these are fast pull ups).
- With proper instructions and supervision one is expected to perform the fast and relaxation phases repeatedly for 5-10 minutes each time for 5 times a day
- Improvement in the exercise should purport one to progress for longer periods of 10-15 seconds and with different positions like standing.
- The ultimate aim is to be able to perform the exercises at other times whenever possible. One need not have to sit on a chair to do these exercises. exercises at other times whenever possible as one need to sit on chair to do the exercise.
- It takes about 3-6 months of regular exercise to notice good improvement with no involuntary loss of urine.

Treatment of Genuine Stress Incontinence

Some of surgery is required to correct the problem causing stress incontinence if pelvic floor exercise is not giving the expected response. If the woman have pelvic organ prolapse this should be treated first before performing surgery for stress incontinence. The primary aim of surgery is to tighten the muscles and structures below the bladder and correct any anatomical displacement.

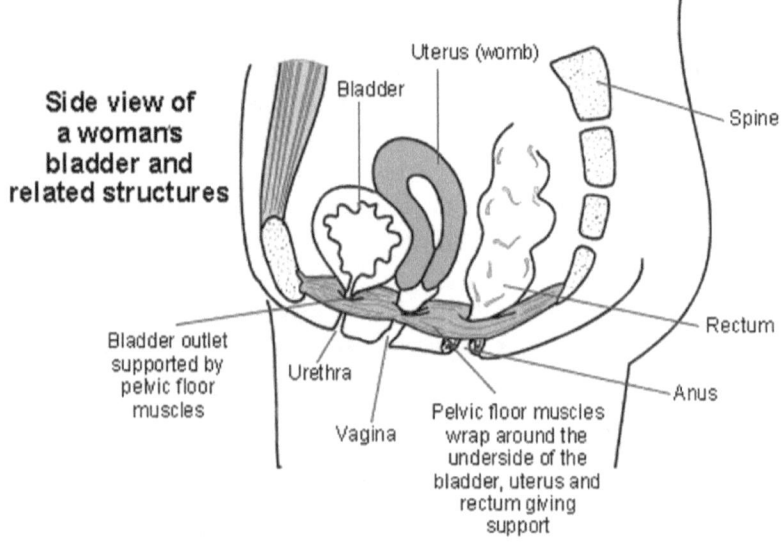

Fig. 22.3 Side view of pelvis showing the pelvic floor support
Source: patient.uk.com

Various procedures may be done to help elevate and hold the lax support tissues around the neck of the bladder (COLPOSUSPENSION). The traditional operation which is called a BURCH COLPOSUSPENSION requires a bikini shaped surgical incision to be made over the lower part of the abdomen just above the level of the bladder. This approach would permit a view of the bladder and the urethra behind thee pubic bone. A few stiches are the placed on the tissues on either side of the neck of the bladder. These stiches are then suspended to the ligaments close to the pelvic bone. The bladder neck is hence elevated and remains so overcoming loss of urine at coughing and sneezing.

Current approaches use the laparoscope to do this procedure as the stay in the hospital is shorter and only key holes are used.

A more popular surgical method is done through the vagina. Tension free tapes are inserted below the urethra and bladder neck effecting a similar outcome i.e elevation of the bladder neck. Tension free tapes operations are preferred as the operative complications are less than the above and success rates are similar.

Women should be counseled that most women remain dry with no stress incontinence after either the BURCH procedure or tension-free-tape but about 10-15 % of women may not totally benefit from the operation. When the procedure does not give the best outcome the procedure may have to be done again or some alternative methods like injection of collagen or silicone materials into the bladder neck (entrance of the bladder) may be done. These are called 'bulking agents' and aim to narrow the opening into the upper part of the urethra. The success rates of the latter, however, are not very encouraging. Artificial sphincters are available as tiny pumps which can be inserted under the bladder neck. This are a rather cumbersome remedy which is not resorted to in most women.

CONCLUSION

Pelvic organ prolapse and urinary incontinence are common gynecological disorders seen in menopausal women. Accurate diagnosis is essential so that appropriate treatment may be suggested. As POP is a form of hernia reconstructive surgery is done. The walls of the vagina that have become lax due to loss of support are strengthened. A hysterectomy is done in those women who are menopausal apart from repair of the vagina. A synthetic material (MESH) is commonly used to give added support when the vagina is repaired.

Symptoms due to urge urinary incontinence and stress incontinence improve with pelvic floor exercise. Medication and lifestyle changes are essential for urge incontinence while a surgical procedure would be advised for stress incontinence. Early consultation and treatment improves quality of life in women with POP and urinary incontinence.

CHAPTER 23

HYSTERECTOMY—
Surgical removal of the uterus

The word HYSTEROS refers to the uterus (womb). Hysteria is a term derived from this word. Hysterectomy refers to surgical removal of the uterus. It is a very common operation worldwide especially in women beyond 40 years. The reasons for removal are numerous. The common conditions that may need hysterectomy are fibroids that are large and cause heavy menstruation, endometriosis that does not respond to conservative medication and partial surgical treatment and of course cancers of the uterus and ovaries. Current concepts in managing heavy menstrual bleeding has questioned the need for hysterectomy contributing to less hospitalization and reduced medical costs. There are many effective drugs that can be used to manage heavy menstrual bleeding without resorting to hysterectomy.

Hysterectomy in the menopausal women may be required if there is precancerous disease or cancer of the genital organs. Prolapse of the uterus is another reason why this procedure is done. The autonomy of women needs to be respected and they should be involved in decision making. The risks and benefits of surgery must be understood before consenting to hysterectomy.

After hysterectomy women must be aware that:

- they can no longer bear children
- they would cease menstruation

At the time of hysterectomy the ovaries are removed if the woman is past menopause or over 50 years. In women who have not attained menopause, removal of the uterus will result in early onset of menopause which may require medical hormone therapy.

HYSTERECTOMY

A knowledge of the anatomy of the internal genital organs helps in understanding the procedure (see Chapter 18). When only the uterus is removed the term HYSTERECTOMY is used. The uterus has a body (corpus) and a neck (cervix). When only the body is removed then a SUBTOTAL HYSTERECTOMY is done. In most cases the body is removed with the cervix (TOTAL HYSTERECTMY). Subtotal hysterectomy is rarely done today.

When the ovaries and fallopian tubes are removed then we use the term SALPINGO-OOPHORECTOMY.

Hysterectomy is done via an incision over the abdomen (bikini incision or a midline incision), through key hole surgery (laparoscopy) or via the vagina. Decision for the approach depends on the disease and expertise available. Following laparoscopic hysterectomy and vaginal hysterectomy patients stay for a shorter time in the hospital and have less post-operative pain.

INDICATIONS FOR HYSTERECTOMY

Prolapse of the uterus is a common reason for vaginal hysterectomy in older women. Very large fibroids may degenerate and cause pain and would have to be removed. Cancer of the uterus (endometrium) is another reason for total hysterectomy. Early cervical cancer can be effectively treated by a more radical hysterectomy that involves not only removal of the uterus but also a quarter of the upper vagina and all the lymph nodes and lymphatic system in the pelvis. Abnormal menstruation may be due to endometrial hyperplasia, some of which may have a potential for transition to cancer of the uterus. Hysterectomy is best done in these cases.

Abnormal bleeding that is only related to a loss of balance of hormones around menopause can be treated with hormones or intrauterine devices that bear progestogen. With impending menopause the problem often abates. Hysterectomy is hence not indicated in most patients with this condition (DYSFUNCTIONAL UTERINE BLEEDING).

The reason ovaries are removed in woman who are above 50 years and require hysterectomy is because of the small risk of development of ovarian tumor if left behind. Ovarian tumors are difficult to detect in the early stages and hence it appears justified removing them after the age of menopause or beyond 50 years.

The issue of routine removal of ovaries between 45-50 years of age is a contentious one. As menopause is inevitable after removal of both ovaries and natural menopause is attained between 48-52 years in most women, one needs to weigh the risks and benefits of OOPHORECTOMY between 45-50 years.

This situation would not arise if the primary problem is not in the uterus but in the ovaries. If a perimenopausal woman has an ovarian tumor past the age of 45 the better option is HYSTERECTOMY AND BILATERAL SALPINGO-OOPHORECTOMY.

Effects of Hysterectomy

A woman who has been menstruating may wonder what happens to her hormone profile should a hysterectomy be done. Myths surrounding this can lead to psychological and psychosomatic ailments especially among the illiterate who presume there will be a hold back of 'bad blood' since the womb has been removed. They need to be made to understand that menstruation only occurs if the uterus is there and if it has been removed no 'bad blood' forms, to begin with. Menstruating women who have a hysterectomy are counseled about early onset of menopause with the procedure especially if the ovaries are also surgically removed well before she is 50 years of age.

Does sexual response decline after hysterectomy? This is related to the attitude to sexual practices as women age. It also depends on the role of the male partner in sexual health. It is difficult to ascribe poor sexual response to hysterectomy alone. It is related to hormonal function particularly to small amounts of androgens. Estrogen withdrawal that is induced with removal of the ovaries together with hysterectomy contributes to dry vagina and atrophic vaginitis. Sexual intercourse is painful if the vagina is dry. Sexual intercourse may be avoided because of personal reasons and atrophic vagina. Appropriate counseling with regards to sexual practices, if desired, can lead to resumption of sexual intercourse after hysterectomy and lead to reasonable sexual happiness.

Vaginal hysterectomy and pelvic floor repair helps to restore the anatomy of the vagina. Healing is complete within two weeks. Sexual intercourse can resume when the woman feels comfortable. Again the use of water based lubricants or local applications of estrogen cream are advised if atrophic vaginitis is a cause of painful intercourse. Regular sexual intercourse prevents narrowing of the vagina. Initial fear of sexual penetration may be avoided by placing a finger or two (lubricated) into the vagina after healing is complete to reassure oneself that sexual intercourse can resume. Such digital exploration prior or sexual intercourse is both reassuring and also contributes to eventual confidence in resumption of sexual activity.

Benefits of Hysterectomy

Women who have suffered from gynecological disorders like chronic pelvic pain, endometriosis, fibroid and prolapse of the uterus will clearly benefit from hysterectomy. Uterine, cervical and ovarian tumors are indications for removal of the uterus (with or without removal of the fallopian tubes and ovaries).

Urinary symptoms are not relieved with hysterectomy and have to be addressed separately. Low backache is a common complaint in the older person and may not be directly related to hysterectomy especially if it is a new complaint. Low backache is not an indication for hysterectomy.

Complications of Hysterectomy

Hysterectomy is a major surgery and can take about an hour or more to perform. The presence of cancer in the genital tract may take a longer time of 2-3 hours. Laparoscopic hysterectomy usually is longer than 'open surgery'. In some gynecological diseases like endometriosis or cancer surgery, careful dissection is required to separate the urinary bladder in front of the uterus and rectum and other parts of the intestine behind before proceeding to excising the uterus and part of the vagina. Inadvertent injury to the bladder, ureter and parts of the intestine is a distant possibility. In cancer surgery additional surgery like removal of a segment of the intestine and fixing a colostomy may be required. If injuries to the bladder, ureter and intestine occur they are fixed at the same sitting. Women are counseled about the possibility of complications prior or surgery.

Blood loss is more in cases of genital cancer surgery as more extensive dissection is needed and blood products may have to be transfused. Again consent would be taken if blood is to be given before surgery especially if the surgery is done as a planned one.

Laparoscopic surgery is known to have other complications like burns and direct injuries with passing of sharp instruments into the abdomen. With skilled surgeons such complications are uncommon. The anesthetist would also be careful in selection of type of anesthesia. Most surgery for laparoscopy requires a general anesthesia where the woman is put to sleep and a tube is passed into the windpipe so as to ventilate her during the procedure. It is possible to administer regional anesthesia in the lower spine when performing gynecological surgery if the surgical approach does not involve laparoscopy.

Some postmenopausal woman may be frail or fraught with various medical ailments which affect the health of the heart and lungs. Such patients need to be evaluated for fitness for anesthesia and will be graded into categories of high and low risk for the procedure.

Following surgery complications like infection of the site of surgery is uncommon but do occur. Urinary infections need to be excluded as many women require a urinary catheter to be inserted prior to, during and even after surgery. Blood clot formation in the veins can lead to THROMBOSIS. If they do occur they need to be urgently treated with blood thinning agents to avoid serious complications of stroke.

Hospitalization

Before planned surgery the woman is examined again by the surgeon and anesthetist. Past history of drug allergy and thrombosis (blood clot) is enquired into. Should she have had blood clots before she would need prophylaxis using anticoagulants like heparin injections? If diabetes mellitus is poorly controlled this needs a review and appropriate treatment before a date for surgery is fixed.

The following tests are routinely done in the older woman:

- Blood and urine tests
- Chest X-ray
- ECG
- Skin preparation and clipping of pubic hair

An informed consent is taken after a thorough explanation is given about the procedure and possible complications. The anesthetist will discuss with the patient about the choice of anesthesia i.e regional or general anesthesia. A urinary catheter would be secured into the urinary bladder prior to surgery. The patient would need to be starved overnight and an intravenous line with fluids is started.

After the surgery the patient is observed in the operation theatre for about an hour to ensure complete recovery from the surgery before being transferred back to the ward. The length of stay in the hospital depends on the type of surgery and reasons for surgery. Cancer patients have extensive dissection and are required to stay longer and the urinary catheter is left for a longer period. Vaginal hysterectomy cases can go home in a day or two. Uncomplicated laparoscopic surgery would require a shorter stay of perhaps 1-2 days.

Recovery after surgery is fairly rapid in the absence of complications. Intravenous fluid infusion is often removed within 1-2 days and the patient is encouraged to sit out of bed and begin ambulating as soon as possible. This ensures good blood circulation in the legs and is a recommended strategy for preventing blood clots. Firm stockinettes are worn for prevention of blood clots in the legs. Most patients who had laparoscopy done would return home much faster as they have less or little pain over the operated site on the skin.

The wound site completely heals within a week of surgery. Movements and early ambulation is encouraged and breathing exercises are continued so as to allow good excursion of the chest wall and lung expansion. This strategy prevents the development of pneumonia, a known complication following general anesthesia.

Special diets are necessary in certain instances where there has been extensive surgery including the removal of segments of the intestines. Most patients who have uncomplicated hysterectomy would be able to tolerate normal food after a couple of days. Passing of wind indicates the gut is moving well and this would give confidence to the patient to resume normal food. Food taboo and food preference after surgery is influenced by cultural and social practices. A normal balanced diet with vitamins and adequate amount of fluids are encouraged before the patient is discharged from hospital.

Medical leave after surgery is given so that the patient can recover and go back to her job. The length of leave given will depend on the disease for which hysterectomy was done. For most benign diseases e.g. fibroid and endometriosis, a shorter leave duration of about 2 weeks is usually sufficient. Following vaginal hysterectomy a similar period of rest ad recovery is suggested. Those who have had laparoscopy and vaginal hysterectomy tend to recover much faster than an abdominal surgery. Cancer patients would require longer leave from work. If additional treatment is given such as radiation therapy and chemotherapy they will have to discuss with their employer and attending doctor about prognosis and potential for return to work.

Medications other than indicated antibiotics and food supplements are not necessary following discharge. Pain relief may be needed for a longer period especially following abdominal surgery in some patients. Hormone therapy may be needed in those with hot flashes and night sweats. Indications for hormones and alternative medication will need consultation.

Sexual Activity

Women may refrain from sexual activity for fear of complications following hysterectomy. Others need time for recovery before they discuss such matters. The indication for surgery would also influence decision as there may a loss of sexual desire or mood. Cancer victims may list sexual activity as low priority. In women desirous of sexual intercourse duration of 4-6 weeks after surgery appears sensible.

Details about use of lubricants and estrogen cream have been discussed in Chapter 21.

Other Activities

Most normal activities can be resumed after about 4 weeks of surgery. Driving and light physical activity is gradually increased over 4-6 weeks as the woman develops confidence and has completely recovered from surgery.

Long Term Follow-up

Most women are seen a month after surgery unless some complication has developed. At the return visit enquiry about general health, resumption of routine work and food consumption is enquired into. Infection of the wound, if it occurs, would have been evident by 7-10 days. The scar over the surgical site should be well healed by this time. A pelvic examination is done to look for complete healing of the vaginal vault. Evidence of urine infection is looked for by asking for symptoms like increased frequency and painful urination. Any uncontrollable loss of urine is also asked for in the event a fistula has developed.

By this time the pathology report of the uterus (and ovaries) would be available and the patient is counseled accordingly.

In cases of cancer like cervical cancer where radical surgery has been done one needs to plan for long term follow up. The pathology report would dictate the completeness of surgery and possible cure. If there is a need for additional treatment like radiation therapy further counseling is given.

CONCLUSION

Hysterectomy is a common surgical treatment done to cure diseases of the uterus and occasionally of the ovaries. It may done through the conventional route by making surgical incisions over the abdomen or vaginally. Laparoscopic surgery is becoming more popular as recovery is faster and hospital stay is shorter. Menopause sets in earlier after hysterectomy and is immediate if the ovaries are removed during hysterectomy. Thorough explanation regarding the indications, procedure and expectations after surgery would help women establish faster adaptation to life after the surgery.

CHAPTER 24

AGING AND MENTAL HEALTH

The confusion between what is normal aging and how it is different from age-related disorders continues to reign when we discuss the aging process and mental health. How do we distinguish cognitive decline from senescence? Gerontology is the study of aging and geriatrics is the study of medical aspects of old age. The subtle difference becomes relevant when we deal with disease and disability. Normal aging refers to aging without pathological aging. There is no illness that is apparent. On the other end of the spectrum is pathological aging when there is severe observable mental deterioration like a person suffering from Alzheimer's disease and has lost touch with the real world. When a person suffers a chronic disease like disabling rheumatoid arthritis she suffers a functional disability that affects her normal aging process. The CDC Centers for Disease Control and Prevention (USA) 2007 states that 80% of those above 65 years will have at least one chronic disease which can be associated with depression. When we use the above definition then it is not difficult to surmise the magnitude of mental health that can potentially affect the aging woman.

Mental health in the older person is different from mental illness. Older people have much lower prevalence of newly diagnosed mental illness like younger ones but do suffer from what is called 'mentally unhealthy days'. About 7% of 65-74 years had mental distress in one report (CDC 2007). Depression is a common symptom of the aging population but this is not part of aging but a mental disorder that is amenable to treatment. Depressive illness can arise from a variety of causes experienced in life as one ages. These may range from co-existing medical disease, lack of social support, stress related dysfunctional disorders and loss of dear ones. This may lead to 'completed' suicide especially in the very old. Completed suicide is a term psychiatrists use to categorize the group that eventually resulted in fatality as compared to those with suicidal thoughts and attempted suicide. Depressive illness and very severe psychological ailment kills about 14.7 per 100000 persons per year after the age of 65 (WHO *2005, Suicide prevention-SUPRE Geneva. Retrieved http:/www. Who.int/mental_health/prevention/suicide.*).

Balancing acts of aging

The concerns of not being able to remember are often linked to aging but this is so wrong. One needs to look at it from several perspectives in coming to terms with our capabilities at a particular age. Experience and wisdom undeniably increase with age. Older persons are often called amateur philosophers. Pragmatic social judgment and expertise in decision making are likeable gains of aging. Skills in thought processes may be retained through the speed of cognitive processing especially when remote memory is recruited though recent memory may decline. As one grows older the social role in the extended family set up is lesser and this could contribute to less need for decision making on important matters. Employability and financial returns decline with retirement, physical and mental disability all of which may be seen in the aging woman. Physical bodily changes in ability to perform tasks and loss of quick responses lowers chances of employability. Taken together, these factors may impact on personality and confidence. This contributes to depressive ailment.

Loneliness, negative views and loss of socialization as a consequence of several factors mentioned are possible targets for directed corrective actions. Customizing the inherent challenges one faces with some degree of optimism is borne by the basic personality structure built over the formative years of life. As one had learnt how to adapt to the numerous obstacles during active adulthood the older or aging adult will find well developed coping mechanisms of yesteryears so useful in confronting and overcoming new challenges. Disappointments and loss of loved ones would have traumatized the young adult and the defense mechanisms learnt would come into force now. Psychological stresses are easier to cope compared to physical disability which could be a permanent feature of aging. When psychological defense mechanisms have been well developed over the years with complete resolution of stressors, it becomes much easier to live with new and emerging stressors. An old friend of mine who had been a widow for the last 10 years and was living by herself was gardening in her limelight years just having gone past 82 years. As we discussed about the life as a 'constant gardener' and if the bad knees she has affected her, she replied," I have learnt to live my life with not a day free of pain. I am not complaining!"

Depressive Illness

It is now known that the commonest ailment woman (and men) will suffer as they grow older is depressive illness. Nearly one fifth of women would have suffered some form of depression throughout their adult lives, especially so after menopause. The Harvard Study of Moods and Cycles recruited women between 36-44 years and followed them up for nine years. Women who were in the transition period were twice as likely to suffer new depressive symptoms as those who had not made the transition to menopause.

The Penn Ovarian Aging Study showed an increase in depressive illness as one went through menopause transition. Two studies involving women in USA and Netherlands also showed higher depressed states in the perimenopausal stage of life. Two factors appear to be associated with these observations i.e higher testosterone level and occurrence of menopause itself.

Problems with sleep in the perimenopausal have been observed to occur in 40-50 % of women. Anxiety, stress, tension and depressive states are implicated. Sleep is disturbed because of hot flashes and night sweats too and there appears to be some relation to hormonal changes i.e estrogen decline and luteinizing hormone increases (that affects the thermoregulatory center in the brain).

Quality of sleep and sleep interruption increases as women age. Apart from the factors mentioned above other factors are changing levels of progesterone and declining melatonin and growth hormone levels in women past 50 years.

Untreated depressive illness contributes to both medical ailment and cognitive decline. It has said that people seek treatment for physical sickness but tend not to report and get appropriate treatment for depressive illness.

Table 24.1 shows the symptoms that should be looked for in making a diagnosis of depression in the older person. A feeling of sadness and unreasonable demands may denote depression and one should seek a medical consult.

Table 24.1. Reported Depressive Symptoms in the Older Person

Memory and Cognitive Function

- Memory loss
- Confusion
- Hallucination
- Delusion (fixed false beliefs)

Social issues

- Social withdrawal

Somatic Symptoms

- Loss of appetite
- Weight loss
- Irritability
- Vague abdominal pains
- Inability to sleep

How can we treat depressive illness in the older person?

The gratifying point is that most persons respond well to treatment which may consist of consultation, counseling, medication, psychotherapy and electroconvulsive therapy. Current approaches to treatment may combine psychotherapy and medication together with a change in surroundings so as to avoid stress factors and loneliness. Old medications like tricyclic compounds and monoamine oxidases are now replaced with the serotonin re-uptake inhibitors (SSRIs) which have less side effects and better tolerability. Electroconvulsive therapy is only prescribed in severe depressive illness on a selected basis. Supportive psychotherapy, group therapy and family therapy are used in treating depressive illness. One of such therapy, Cognitive-behavior therapy, is described. Treatment has to be individualized and tailored to the cause of depression.

Cognitive-behavior model

Maladaptive behavior is due to beliefs and thoughts that are wrong. Our mind is filled with negative emotions. The brain is convinced that what is going though the mind is by far the best way of coping. However, the person knows this displeases her. Such a way of thinking needs to be altered by taking alternative approaches. This is what the cognitive behavior model refers to.

Behavior of an individual is influenced by several factors. There are certain expectations and modes of response that are evoked. These have been internalized over the years. The cognitive-behavior model uses a combination of exploring the mind to determine maladaptive behavior and to suggest alternative yet positive approaches so that the thinking mechanism changes to make it more pleasant. This whole process needs a period of engagement with a counselor and is based on how learning occurs in the mind.

To put in simple terms some emotional response that is expressed as a result of an event occurs as such not because of the event itself but as to how the mind interprets it. There is a distortion of thoughts and evoked responses and the strategy is to work on such skewed interpretations to make good what is wrong.

The process is summarized below in a 'cartoon form'

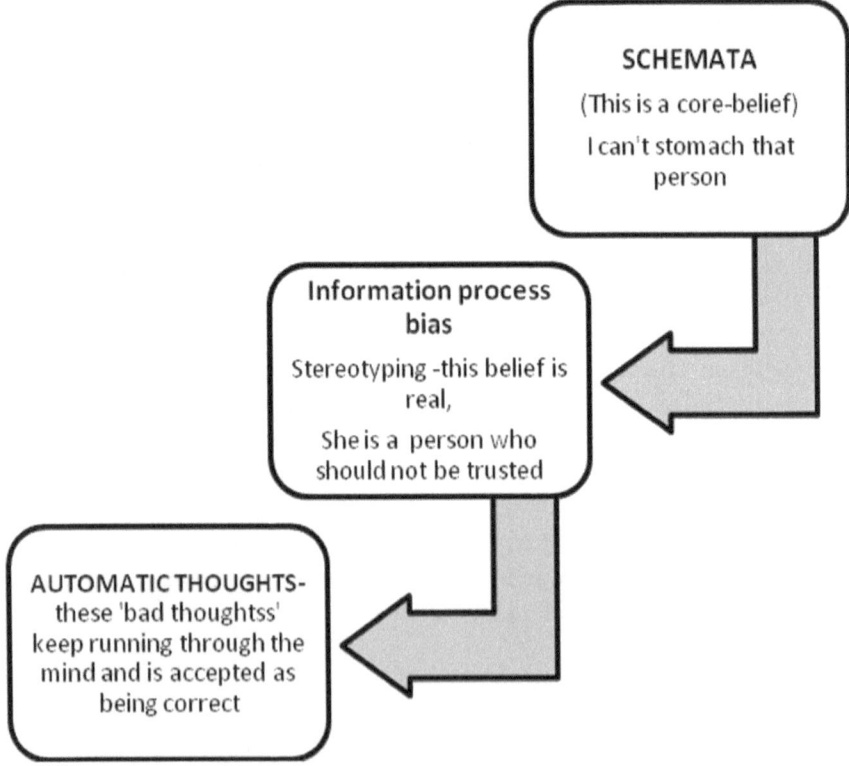

Fig. 24.1: The Cognitive-Behavior Model

Clearly if the person has internalized such a thought about a particular person or she will sustain the 'wrong concept', that which is the cause of her mental discomfort. Unless this maladaptive behavior is changed one will continue to experience the discomfort when such similar events recur. Core beliefs were wrong to start with and more rational thinking has to be learnt. This would be the only way to get out of one's misery. Positive thinking and changed behavior cannot occur with explanation alone but needs formal counseling by experts in this area such as psychologists and professional counselors.

How do we keep our mind fit?

We have several methods in keep the body fit. We have been advised on the importance of maintaining our weight lest we become obese, keep the cholesterol down and treat diabetes if we have this metabolic disease. We can also keep our mind fit by various stimulating exercises. An idle mind leads to lethargy and disinterest. Mentally challenging exercises have been shown to increase the brain circuits. Doing the daily jig-saw puzzle and cross-word puzzle stimulates intellect. Reading a book or writing 500 words a day has been recommended as ways to stimulate the brain. Numerous on-line brains stimulating games are available for those who are computer-savvy (www.memoryfitnessinstitute.org/default.asp). The WHO report (2000) on Intellectual Disability and Ageing highlights the need for a comprehensive network of support and facilities for the aging person and this material makes useful reading.

Stress reduction is clearly a much needed strategy as undue stress is harmful to both physical and mental health. Periods of stress causes intense internal conflict and disturbs our ability to think rationally. In fact if is true that the chemical products that are released during stress influences both thinking and learning, memory can also be affected. As stress is harmful one needs to develop strategies to overcome stress. Sharing views with others and finding a person to talk about stressful events is simple and useful. Exercises and relaxation, reading a book and avoiding being alone are effective measures. Some have found solace in writing about personal matters in magazines while others need the services of counsellors and psychologists. Getting out of the usual routines and joining the local 'tai chi' morning exercise group are good and cheap means of overcoming many 'stressors'.

The John Hopkins's Health Alert Bulletin reports that regular exercise reduces cognitive decline by 60% and vascular related dementia by 50%. A nice program on stress management was shown on Discovery Health Channel and is worth accessing at health.discovery.com/centres/stress/stress.html.

Digital technology has been both a boost and a bane to society but has promoted living at home for the old easier as they are able to access both information and help with the use of communications much faster and better. Reminders for daily living can be programmed and many older people are able to stay home with little help from children and minders. Living in familiar surroundings when there is cognitive decline causes less stress and promotes confidence. Staying connected with friends and family is easier with current communication tools like the face book and face time. Loneliness is kept at bay through modern digital technology. With wisdom comes intellectual thinking and the need to explore more. Many older people find more time to ponder over life and cosmology. They find the need to explore spiritualism and meditation to reduce stress and remain connected to new friends and society at large. The comfort derived from spirituality and support can bring meaning to life and one begins to look at the brighter renewed interest.

Guidelines in promoting older people's mental well being focussing on occupational therapy (National Institute of Clinical Excellence in UK (2008) on Physical Activity) draws attention to a program that encourages exercise as a routine. This is summarised in Table 24.2.

Table 24. 2 Suggested Exercise Program for Good Mental Health

▪ Establish daily routines which addresses nutrition and attention to personal care
▪ Community based physical exercise programmes tailored to individuals (swimming, walking, dancing)—resistance training, stretching and toning
▪ Exercise for 30 minutes a day five days a week (can be broken into 10 minute bursts)
▪ Participation in local walking schemes to improve mental health (consider mobility of individual)
▪ Seek advice of occupational therapists to tailor to individual's needs

*Adapted from NICE Guidelines (http://guidance.nice.org.uk/PH16)

Memory and Memory Loss

The commonest complaint as one grows older is forgetfulness. We forget the name of the movie we saw the previous month and we can't locate the car keys. This loss of memory frustrates us and we try to compensate by following some routines. Always hang the key in the same place and do not let others re-arrange your personal items. You use alarms to remind you when to take the medication and use daily dispensers to ensure you do not forget the frequency and types of medication to be taken.

The hippocampus is a tiny part of the brain that is largely involved in retaining and retrieving information that we receive and this specialised centre becomes less efficient in its function as one ages. Other factors that have been implicated in memory loss are less efficient absorption of vital nutrients for this specific brain function and not enough of 'brain food' being available because of altered nutrition for various reasons. There is also a programmed decline in certain growth hormones and also specific proteins which are essential in brain cell protection and repair. Less efficient blood flow to the brain due to aging and diseased lining of the blood vessels can impair oxygenation and nutrient transfer leading to memory loss and declines in cognitive functions.

Loss of memory of a temporary nature occurs in women who have poorly controlled diabetes and develop metabolic complications and dehydration. This can cause confusion and stupor and requires urgent treatment. Medication like insulin can cause low blood sugars resulting in confusion and even coma. The older woman is not able to metabolise medication as well as the young and levels of the drugs tend to build up causing undesired side effects including memory loss. Care should be taken when prescribing antihistamines, anti-depressive and anti-anxiety medication to older people. Often lower doses would be required. Depression is associated with loss of memory and so is alcohol abuse and nutrient deficiencies like Vitamin B 12.

Strategies to overcome memory loss

Memory loss does not equate to dementia but is part of aging. Active steps need to be taken to compensate for such forgetfulness so as not to be overwhelmed by these events. It is not true that we can remember everything in daily life especially with the information overload and the bombardment of information by media. Many old people develop good strategies that help them to cope with daily routines. Some has been mentioned above. Following routines helps a great deal. Staying in the same environment makes them feel safe and helps them follow routines. The use of calendars, diaries and smart phones are of great help. Jotting down daily tasks and events takes the stress off the mind. They say that writing the tasks down promotes retention as visual memory is superior to other modes. Learning new things can be challenging but helps in building memory. Try joining an adult class and you see purpose in it. Apart from meeting people from all walks of life there will be motivation and drive to learn new skills and mastery of such skills not only is beneficial to you but adds to the confidence you need. Learning is improved by associations and use of analogies. Inability to recall is often one aspect of memory that embarrasses us and one should not be frustrated by this. Should you not be able to recall a particular information, work at it for awhile and say to yourself it will come back. Look it up in the internet and overcome the frustration.

The American Medical Association has published a comparative table that distinguishes normal aging and dementia and it is worth looking up (http://www.ama-assn.org/ama1/pub/upload/mm/433/aging_vs_dementia.pdf). Basically in dementia there is a loss of touch with the real world. Normal aging shows evidence of independent existence and complaints of memory loss. The demented person requires assistance in performing normal activities of the day and would only state that there is loss of memory when specifically questioned. The family notices a marked decline in the dementia as there is loss of words and expressivity of thought. Often one loses one's way around whether at home or outside. There is social isolation in dementia, a sense of exclusion and apathy and one is unable to learn new tasks or perform known tasks. There are mental tests that can be used to evaluate the degree of dementia. Dementia is often slow in onset and the decline in cognitive functions is gradual. Problem solving is near impossible as is following a conversation.

Conclusion

Mental health is of concern as one grows older. With aging comes a variety of psychological problems emanating from the environment and family relations. Employability becomes difficult and physical disability may contribute to immobility. As most women beyond 65 years would have at least one chronic disease this can contribute to depressive illness especially when there are medical complications. Aging is also related to some degree of memory loss but intact coping mechanisms can improve quality of life. Depressive illness can be troubling but most are treatable. Support groups in the community can do a great deal in addressing the mental health of older persons and so can the family by engaging them in cavities that would benefit the individuals and society.

Dementia is not aging but a distinct neurological disorder and needs to be evaluated and managed with empathy and rehabilitation. Regular exercise, good nutrition and a safe environment can promote mental health in the older woman.

Useful Resources

1. Older People: Mental Health Foundation. http://www.mentalhealth. org.uk/help-information/mental-health-a-z/O/older-people/ retrieved on 29 July 2013
2. Mental Health in: The Healthy Women pp 207 http://www.women shealth.gov/publications/our-publications/the-healthy-woman/ mental_health.pdf retrieved on 29 July 2013
3. Fawcett B, Reynolds J. Mental Health and Older Women: The challenges for social perspectives and community capacity building. British Journal of Social Work 2010: 40(5): 1488-1502

BIBLIOGRAPHY

Beyene Y. Cultural significance and physiological manifestations of menopause: a biocultural analysis. Culture Med Psychiatric 1980; 10:47-71

Colditz GA, Stampfer MJ, Willet WC. Prospective study of estrogen replacement therapy and risk of breast cancer in postmenopausal women. JAMA 1990; 264:2648-53

DuPont WD, Page DL. Menopausal estrogen replacement therapy and breast cancer. Arch Intern Med 1991; 151:67-72

Flint M. The Menopause: reward or punishment? Psychosomatics. 1975:15:161-63

Greene JG, Cooke DJ. Life stress and symptoms at the climacteric. Br J Pschol 1981:136:486-91

Heany RP. Calcium, bone health and osteoporosis. In Peck WA (Ed). Bone and Mineral 1990; 11:67-84

Konsensus om bruk av estrogen og etter overgansaldern. Nov 27-29, 1990. Distributed by Norwegian Research Council, Oslo, Norway.

Kansi JA, Passmore R. Calcium supplementation of the diet—II BMJ.1989; 298:205-8

Krall EA, Dawson HB. Walking is related to bone density and rates of bone loss. Is J Med 1994; 96:20-26?

Macintyre I, Stevenson JC, Whitehead MI. Calcium for prevention of postmenopausal bone loss. Lancet 1988 (i): 900-2

Melton LR. Screening for osteoporosis. Ann Int Med 1990; 112:516-28

Menopause-Live Well-NHS Choices.www.nhs.uk/live well/menopause

Ponay N, Hamoda H, Arya R, Savvas M. The 2013 The British Menopause Society & Women's Health Concern recommendations on Hormone Replacement Therapy. Menopause Int 2013; doi:10.117/175404531.3489645

Riggs ML. Melton LJ. Involutional osteoporosis. NEJM 1986; 314:1676-86

Sandilyan MB, Dening T. Mental health around and after menopause. Menopause Int.2011;17(4):142-147. doi:10.1258/m.2011.011102

Sivalingam Nalliah. Living with Cancer. Pelandok Publication 1993. Kuala Lumpur

Stampfer MJ. A prospective study of The Menopause 1988. Oxford Blackwell Scientific Publishers. London

Studd JWW, Collins WP. Estradiol and testosterone implants in the treatment of psychosexual problems in postmenopausal women. Br J Obstet Gynecol 1977; 84: 314-1319

The 2012 Hormone Therapy Position Statement of the North American Menopause Society. Menopuase Int 2012;19(3):257-271.doi:10.1097/gme.Ob013.31824b970a